St. Louis State Hospital:

A 150-YEAR JOURNEY TOWARD HOPE

Amanda Hunyar

Reedy Press
PO Box 5131
St. Louis, MO 63139
www.reedypress.com

Library of Congress Control Number: 2019931714

ISBN: 9781681062082

Printed in the United States of America
19 20 21 22 23   5 4 3 2 1

Dedication

This book is dedicated to past, present, and future clients.

and

To Dr. Louis Hirsch Kohler who dedicated his life to the service of his patients, his staff, and his country.

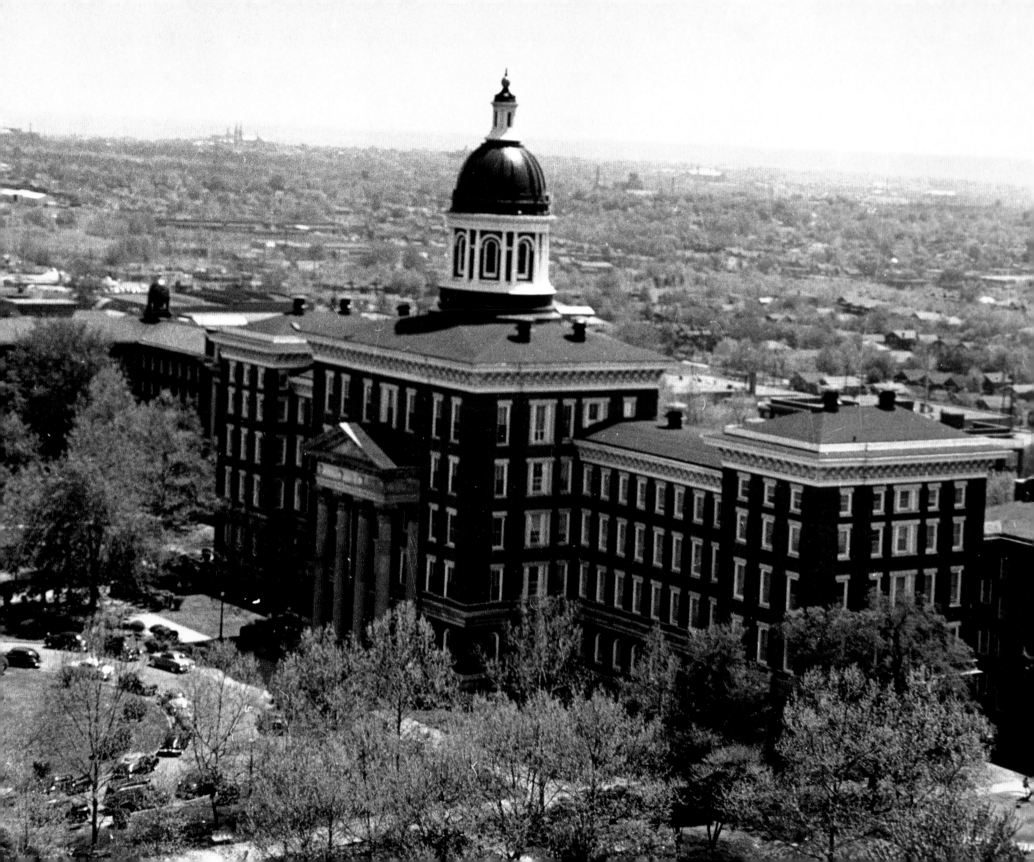

St. Louis State Hospital:
A 150-YEAR JOURNEY TOWARD HOPE

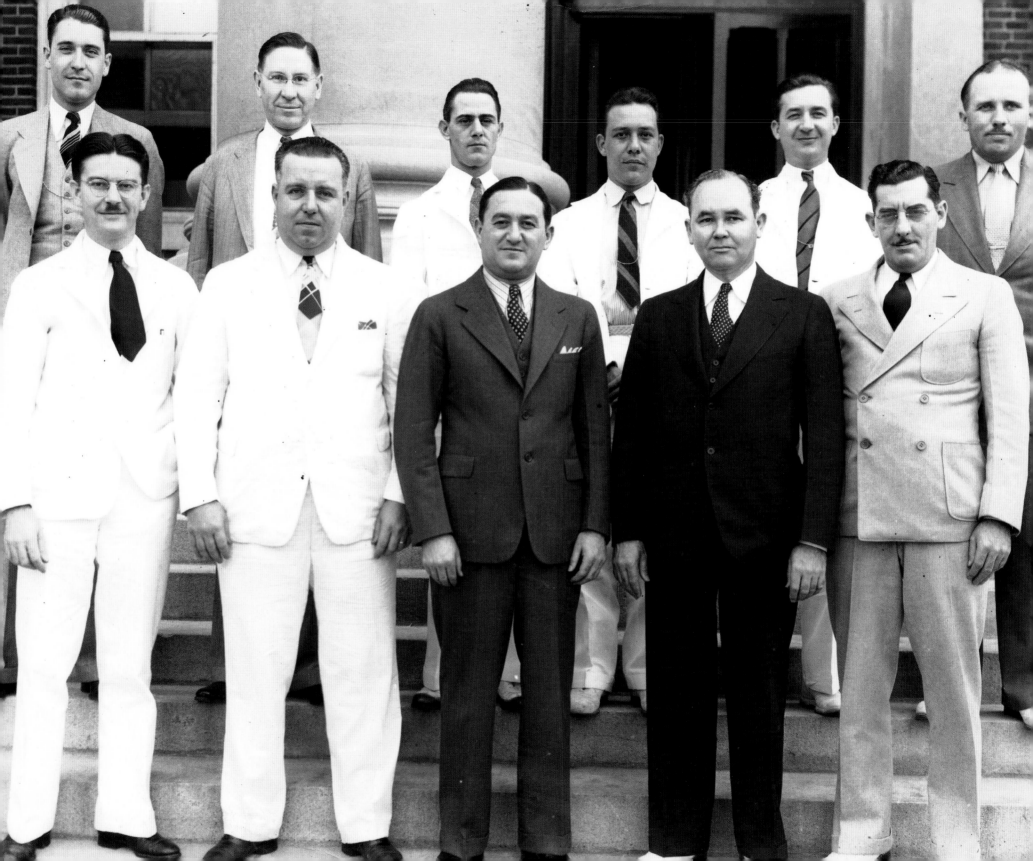

Acknowledgments

The author would like to thank all of those who provided support and encouragement during this project. Special recognition for amazing research skills to Mike Everman, Rena Schergen, Sabrina Gorse, Emily Jaycox, Dennis Northcott, Bob Moore, Linda Chestnut, Scott Clark, Tonya Hays-Martin, Judy Schmitt, Ann Zolla, Andrea Pfaff, Susie Anderson-Bauer, and everyone in special collections at St. Louis Public Library. Thank you to the Auxiliary for all you do and to Helping Hands for funding. Finally, to my family. All of you.

"Early and proper treatment of the nervous diseases will, in many instances, stay the development of insanity, which alone would give the suggested sanitarium its raison d'etre." —Dr. Runge, 1903

Contents

"Our task consists in attempts at restoration of the afflicted human mind to its normal function whenever feasible, and in efforts to stay further deterioration when a return to pristine integrity is made impossible." —Dr. Runge, 1903

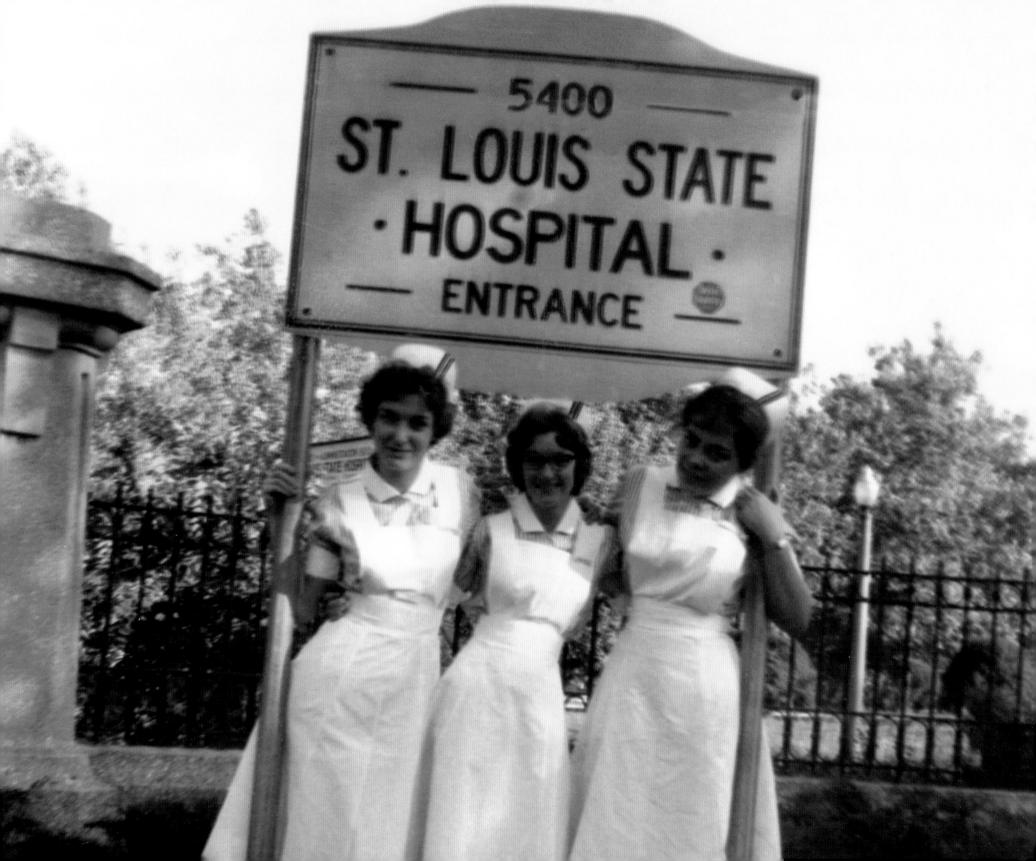

Foreword

I have had the unique privilege of serving in a leadership capacity at two of Missouri's most historic institutions during their respective sesquicentennial celebrations: Fulton State Hospital in 2001, and St. Louis Psychiatric Rehabilitation Center in 2019. Such moments require one to reflect upon the evolution in the care of individuals with mental illness. This includes our history of noble aspirations to treat, even to cure, in the hope that we can rid individuals of psychiatric illness that robs them of their youth, their promise, their connection to family, and a life worth living. We must also confront our darker history, our views of the "lunatic," and other stigmatizing sobriquets too cruel to mention, that have been used to justify society's efforts to rid itself of individuals judged too damaged, too dangerous, or just too painful to bear in its midst.

St. Louis Psychiatric Rehabilitation Center has been integral to that history and to mental health service delivery in the greater St. Louis region for 150 years. This was true in its initial incarnation in 1869 as the St. Louis County Insane Asylum, when nothing but grassland surrounded the hospital; or as the name changed to the St. Louis City Insane Asylum when the city's boundaries crept westward and the Hill neighborhood grew up around it. It remained true when the city fathers deeded it to the State of Missouri in 1948 as St. Louis State Hospital, the name by which it has been known for most of its history; or in the hospital's current form since 1997 as a modern psychiatric rehabilitation center. It has been true when it operated 300 beds at its founding, or 4,400 beds in the 1950s, or the 180 beds it has today. It was true whether the hospital provided a full spectrum of psychiatric services to all individuals with mental disorders, needing treatment that ranged from acute to chronic, from child to geropsychiatry, from outpatient to emergency room, or whether it provided a more specialized focus on those with a serious and persistent mental illness in need of court mandated long-term treatment.

In its one and a half centuries, this hospital has walked with its patients along a difficult and meandering path, aiding them as they carefully picked their way between the razor's edge separating optimism from despair, and illness from health. In its efforts to be of help, and in past ignorance of the causes of mental illness and modern forms of treatment available only today, the hospital—like all other psychiatric facilities of its age—has occasionally stumbled, sometimes offering only long-term institutionalization, if not outright detention, or providing "treatments" that did more harm than good. But more often than not, it has meant succor and support. This was so from its first beginnings, in what was known as the "Moral Model," in which patients were given the opportunity to rest and recuperate in the countryside, participating in pastoral and restorative work, while living with caregivers who treated them like family, and above all, with dignity and respect. It is certainty so today, with the hospital offering scientifically formulated and evidence based practices that enable its patients to better manage their illness and safely reintegrate back into society, with the chance to live, love, work, and play that the rest of us take for granted. The path has been long, and not without missteps, but it has been fruitful 150 year journey toward hope, a journey replete with the promise of an even brighter future.

Felix T. Vincenz, Ph.D.
Chief Operating Officer

County Insane Asylum, rear view 1869

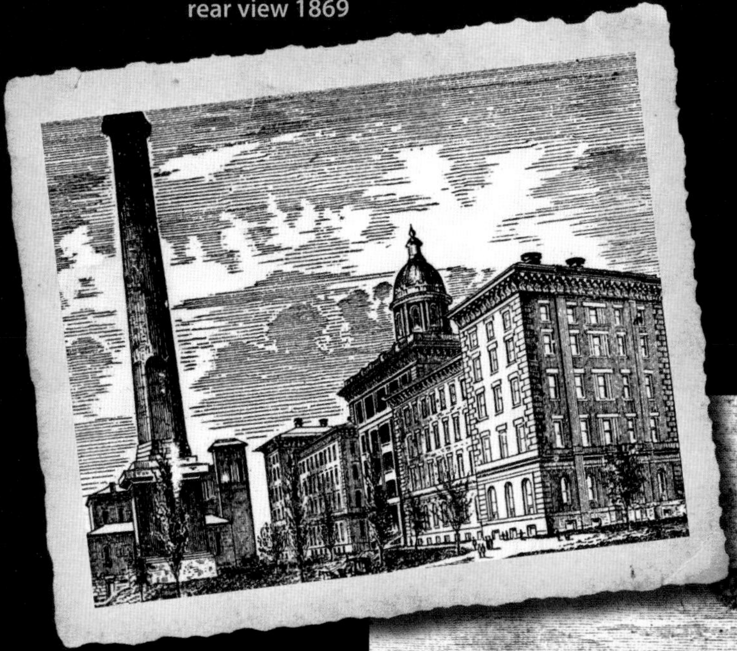

Rumbold's Legacy

Soon after the asylum was approved, county architect William Rumbold set to work. Rumbold's work could be seen throughout St. Louis, with the most notable example housing the very court that passed legislation for the new building. The courthouse, located in the heart of the city, was highlighted by the large dome and decorative rotunda. With these features in mind, Rumbold decided to incorporate the grandeur of the courthouse into the hospital scheme.

1869

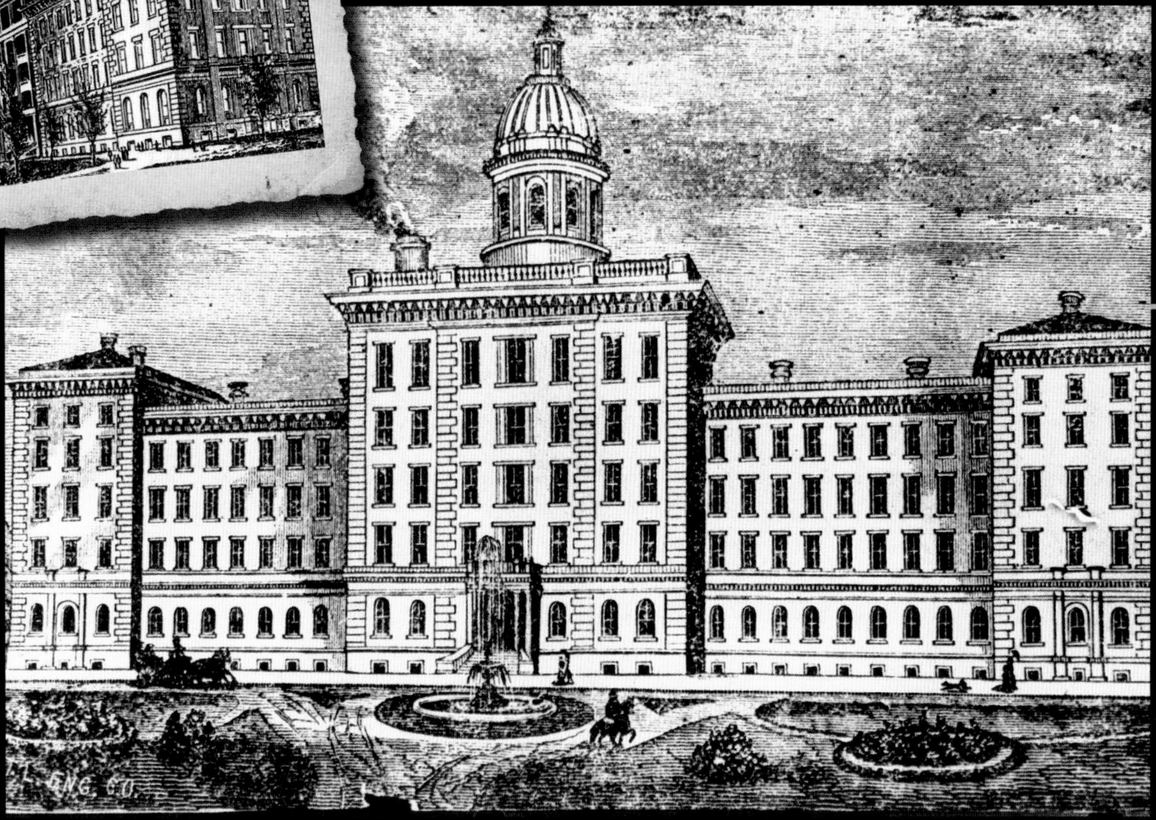

Architect's rendering, 1869

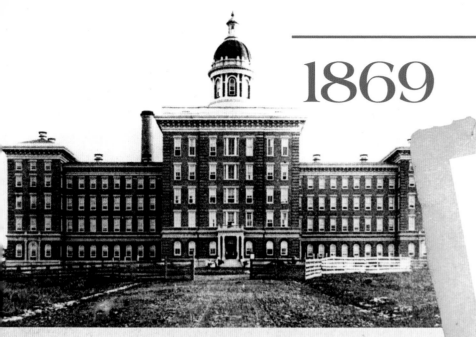

1869

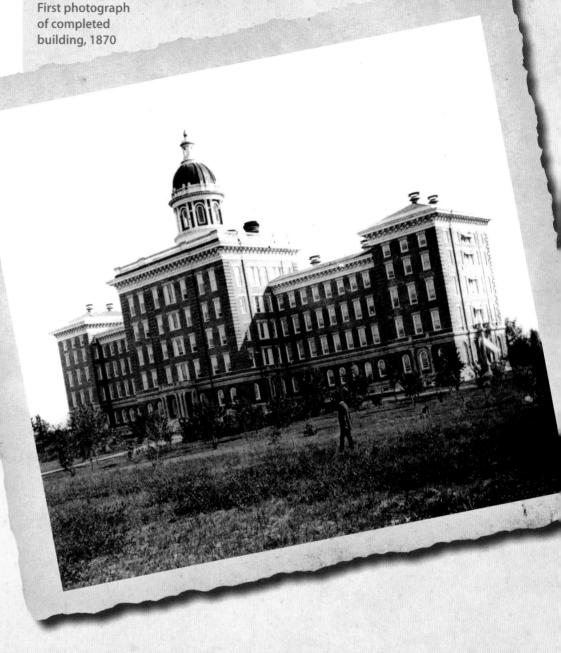

First photograph of completed building, 1870

Final Product

Modified due to cost as well as available land, Rumbold's version called for a center structure of five floors flanked by two wings of four floors. Each wing ended in a five-floor tower. The cast-iron dome sat atop the center section and was supported by a series of circular rooms that repeated floor by floor to the basement. The first four floors of the towers served as day rooms. The top floor of each tower contained spacious living quarters for the resident physicians and their families.

Despite funding shortages, the completed building remained reasonably true to the original plan, although it was left to sit on a mostly bare patch of earth. Fortunately, help came when community leader Henry Shaw donated more than two hundred shade trees of different varieties.

Photograph from 1872 featuring shade trees from Henry Shaw

1872

Atwood's Attitudes 1832–1917

For all their respective stubbornness, Dr. Stevens and Dr. Howard had proven themselves to be progressive in their social stances. In particular, they demonstrated a commitment to moral treatment for all patients, regardless of illness or race. These beliefs were spread throughout the household and were expected to be followed by all staff. This enlightened view would be sorely tested under Dr. LeGrand Atwood.

Atwood came of age as pre-Civil War tensions were escalating. Firmly on the side of the Confederacy, he joined the raid against abolitionist John Brown in Kansas. Shortly after, he signed up with the South as a captain. Unfortunately for Atwood, his time defending the Confederacy was cut short when he was captured after the Battle of Dry Wood Creek in 1861. Political influence secured his release and return to his home in Marshall, Missouri; his refusal to pledge allegiance to the Union, however, led to his banishment. He and his family settled in the St. Louis suburb of Ferguson, where he began practicing medicine.

His political connections and leadership abilities eventually led to his appointment as superintendent in 1887. He dedicated a section of his first annual report to the "Insanity of Negroes." According to Atwood, the "acquisition of freedom" of former slaves contributed a "vastly disproportionate" number of insane compared with the Caucasian race. In his opinion, social equality in the world was "impossible, unattainable, and undesirable"; therefore, it should be no different inside the asylum. He demanded the establishment of segregated wards as soon as possible, but the lack of space kept this from becoming a reality. His outlook on other topics, such as epilepsy and the female gender, was similarly harsh.

Atwood was considered a grand orator and eloquent writer. These skills, combined with his contacts in city society, secured the funding for several repair projects. Likewise, he was able to increase community involvement, including the addition of several forms of entertainment such as "magic lantern shows." He resigned from the superintendent's post in 1891 to focus on his career. He returned to private practice and eventually became mayor of Ferguson.

LeGrand Atwood

Stevens vs. Howard

As the population of St. Louis spread outward to the county, rumblings of discontent foreshadowed the infamous split of 1876. The plan officially separating St. Louis City and St. Louis County into two entities with two governments was known as the Scheme and Charter. The asylum, originally built in the county but controlled by members in the city, found itself in a tug of war.

Under the Scheme and Charter, Dr. Howard was superintendent, having been appointed by the city court. Due to the asylum's location, though, the county court decided to take possession of the building and its inhabitants. In order to make the transition swift and painless, the county judges called Dr. Stevens from retirement and appointed him superintendent. Dr. Stevens, having already served in the position as well as being a prominent member of society, would ease the asylum through the adjustment phase until full county control was established. No one, however, was prepared for Dr. Howard's reaction to all this.

Self-described as a "loyal servant" to the city court and mayor, Dr. Howard dug in his heels and refused to vacate the premises, even as Dr. Stevens set up camp, literally, on the grounds. The dueling superintendents each submitted the usual reports on asylum conditions to their respective authorities. Local newspapers got involved when Howard and Stevens began writing editorials aimed at one another.

The situation came to a head on February 1, 1877, when a group of fed-up judges from the county court rustled up a gang of toughs from Butchertown and headed up to the asylum. The plan was simple: one of the judges would knock on the front door, and when Howard answered, the Butchertown boys would pull him out of the building. The judges would enter the building, lock out Howard, and physically install Stevens.

Again, everyone had underestimated Howard and his connections. Already planning for the worst, Howard had amassed his own gang consisting of loyal hospital staff, police officers, and friends. When the fateful knock came, Captain Fox of the Mounted Police answered the door. Taken aback, the judges mumbled an excuse that they wanted to see how Dr. Howard and Dr. Stevens were getting along. Fox replied that he didn't know about Stevens, but Howard was "bully." With that he let out a whistle, and Howard's supporters appeared from "up through the floor, out of the cracks in the walls, and fell from the chandeliers and all conceivable places." The Howard men were armed and ready to fight. Sensing the odds, the Butchertown boys headed home quickly, followed by the judges as fast as they could get their horses to run.

Eventually the county court decided—no doubt influenced by Howard's stubbornness—to cede control to the city. Dr. Stevens headed back to his home none the worse for wear.

Dr. Charles Stevens

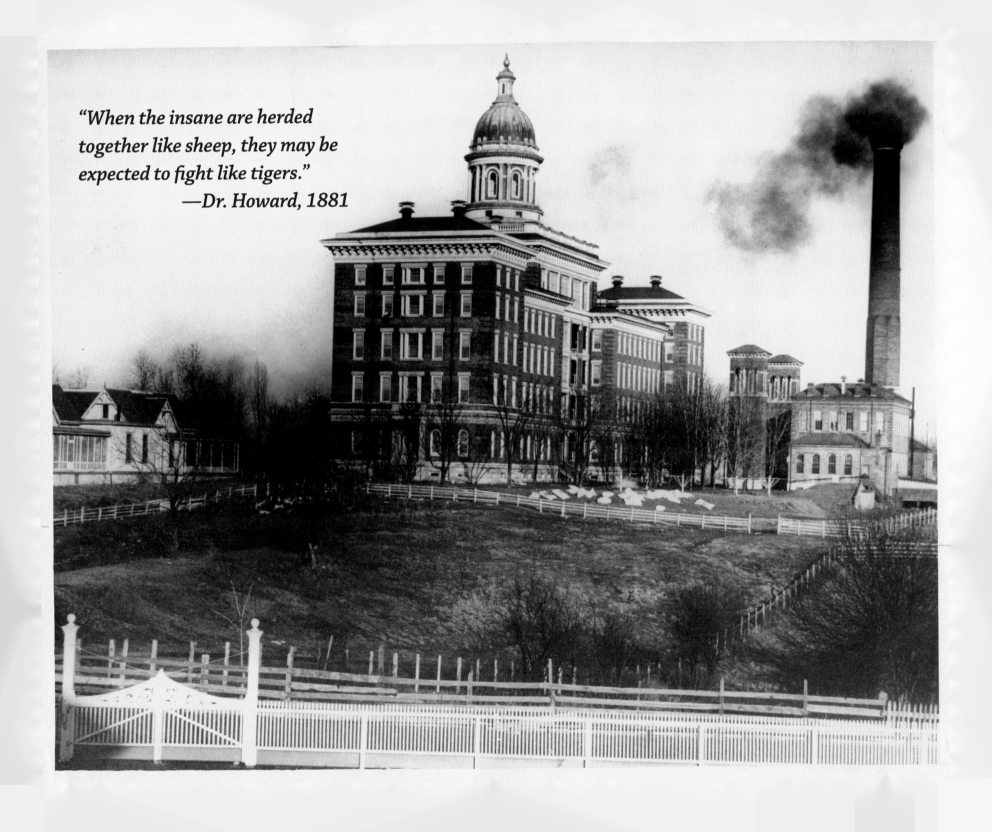

"When the insane are herded together like sheep, they may be expected to fight like tigers."
—Dr. Howard, 1881

Dr. Edward C. Runge

Edward Charles Runge came to St. Louis by way of St. Petersburg, Russia, in the early 1880s. Always scientifically minded, he attended St. Louis Medical College, graduating with his degree in 1891. By 1895 his reputation as a compassionate and ethical professional led to his appointment as superintendent of the asylum.

Upon taking the assignment, Dr. Runge sought to return the overcrowded building to its roots as a household. He insisted that all staff put themselves in the proverbial shoes of their patients. One of his first priorities was to learn the name and history of each patient. Soon after, he implemented a variety of entertainments and diversions to fill the patients' days. Large groups of patients would wander the grounds and traverse Tower Grove Park. Higher-functioning female patients would be taken on shopping trips to downtown department stores. Those without resources were provided funds from Dr. Runge's own pocket.

Mrs. Runge opened up the superintendent's apartment for afternoon tea and evening readings. Well-behaved patients could spend hours with the couple reciting poetry and listening to music. These incentives, which appeared to be successful, were used in place of restraints to encourage appropriate behaviors. Reports of the time show a decrease in the use of mechanical and chemical restraints.

Runge's leadership took the asylum into a new century. His beloved patients were able to attend such delights as the 1904 World's Fair and the opening of the new downtown library. He published numerous papers on the successes and failures of his time in office. He was quick to praise and, unfortunately, just as quick to call out corrupt behavior. His well-written missives caught the attention of city politicians, and he was eventually ousted from office.

He refused to leave without a fight, but the battle left him weary and in ill health. Four months after he resigned, he died of pneumonia. His friends and admirers believed a broken heart and spirit hastened his demise.

"In spending our days among them, we must be like the very sunshine to them, cheering and inspiring them with that essential element of human happiness—hope."
—Dr. Runge, 1901

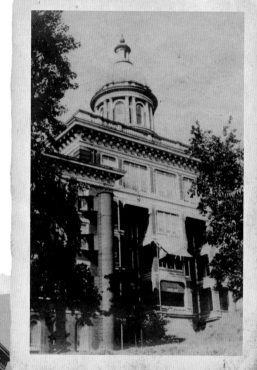

East Wing, rear view, 1876

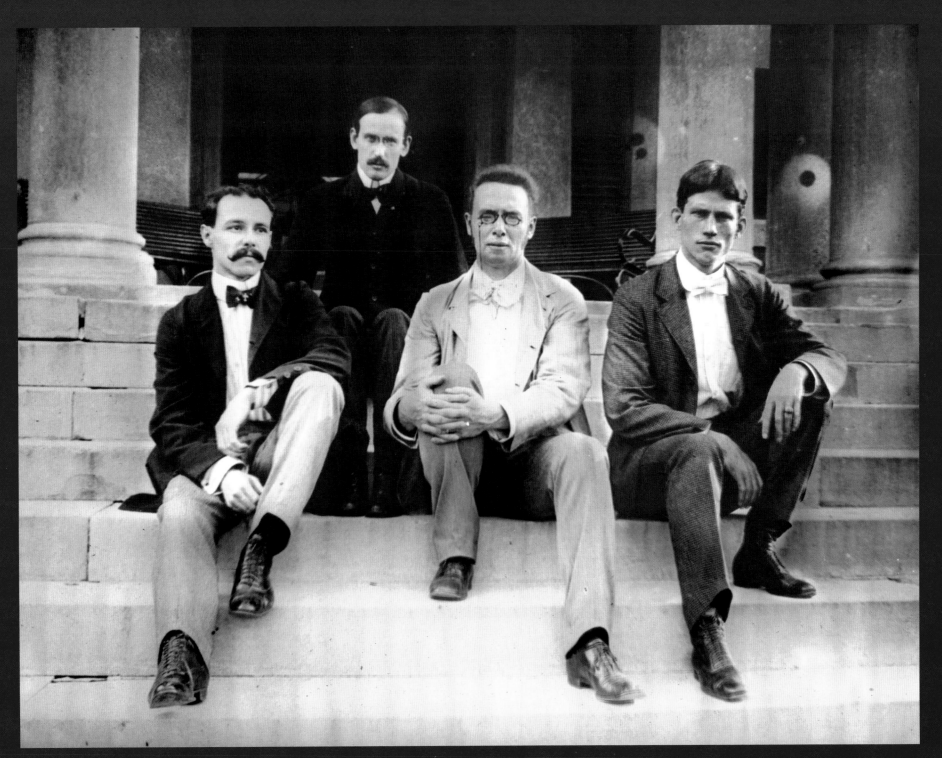

Reasons to be Admitted

Contrary to urban legend, being admitted to the asylum was more difficult than showing up at the door with the "afflicted" in tow. In the early years, admittance to the hospital was only allowed at the discretion of the court. Sufficient evidence had to be presented along with the petition, and more often than not cases were dismissed. By the mid-1880s hospital administration had the discretion to refuse or accept as they saw fit, but overcrowded conditions meant that they were judicious in those they took in. Even then, it was possible for the doctors to change their mind depending on further analysis of the patient. It was not unheard of, for example, for someone guilty of a crime to fake insanity in order to avoid jail.

That being said, for those who were admitted, the reasons given varied according to the medical knowledge of the time as well as societal norms and occupations. In 1869 "War Excitement" accounted for several admissions. The late 1870s and 1880s saw many patients with "Unrequited Affection, Domestic Unhappiness, and Spiritualism." At the turn of the century, reasons for admission began to reflect more scientific reasoning. "Saturnismus Chronic" (chronic lead poisoning), "Delirium of Septicaemia" (blood poisoning), and "Lues Cerebralis" (childhood syphilis) were all listed. By the mid-twentieth century, more recognizable terms such as "Manic Depression," "Dementia," and "Schizophrenia" were being used.

TABLE NO. 5.

FORMS OF DERANGEMENT.

FORMS OF DERANGEMENT.	From April 23d, 1869, to April 23d, 1874.			From April 23d, to September 1st	
	Males.	Females.	Total.	Males.	Females.
Acute Mania	68	71	139	1	1
Chronic Mania	65	70	135	12	10
Melancholia	32	29	61	1	4
Dementia	55	54	109	2	1
Methomania	36	5	41	2	
Puerperal Mania		27	27		3
Hysteria		3	3		
Acute Periodical Mania	6	6	12		1
Recurrent Mania	3	6	9		1
Mcnomania	14	9	23		
Mental Imbecility	7	7	14		
Paresis	4		4		
Epileptic Mania	10	32	42	2	
Chronic Periodical Mania	2	2	4		
Mania Sine Delirio	1	1	2		
Dementia Epileptica	10	6	16		
Dementia Senilis	1	9	10		
Idiocy	5	7	12	2	2	4
Pathomania	2	1	3		
Delirium	1		1		
Erotomania	1		1		
Not Insane	6	2	8		
TOTALS.	329	347	676	22	23	45

St. Louis State Hospital

TABLE 5-A. MENTAL DISORDERS OF ALL ADMISSIONS, ALL DISCHARGES, ALL DEATHS, ALL CASES IN RESIDENCE, AND ALL CASES OUT ON JUNE 30, 1950, BY STATUS OF ADMISSION AND SEX—Continued

211

Reasons for admissions 1880s and 1950s

A Tribute to Miss Wolff

The following poem was discovered by an amateur historian in 1989. It had been written in the cover of a cookbook. While the author remains anonymous, according to Dr. Runge's 1899 annual report, Miss Wolff was employed as a "Night Watch" attendant.

CITY INSANE ASYLUM, ST. LOUIS MO

The Asylum stands on a beautiful height,
From all sides at a distance it comes in sight.
The stars and stripes float in the breeze,
The grounds are shaded by many trees.

In the morning the ladies who have kept watch at night,
Are replaced by the attendants who see that all is right.
The attendants whom I have seen were kind to me,
In all truth some were as kind as kind could be.

It is curious to see the patients when they go out to walk,
Some of them are sullen and silent, others like to talk,
Some are cursing and swearing while others try to pray,
Many are talking of nonsense and don't know what they say.

Many thanks Miss Wolff for all your kindness unto me,
I hope God will reward you throughout eternity.
Please have an intention for me when at prayer,
I promise in return in mine you'll have a share.

—May 17, 1899

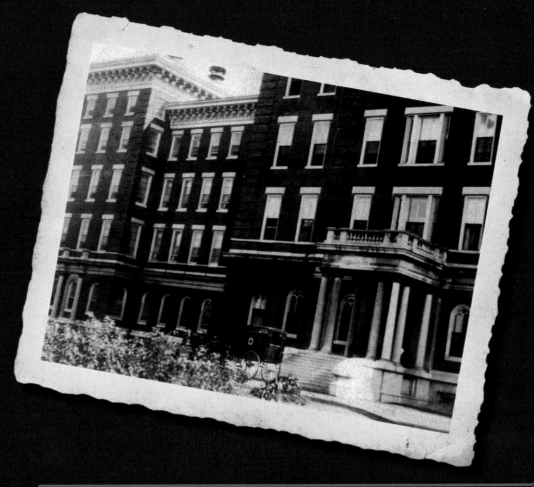

1899

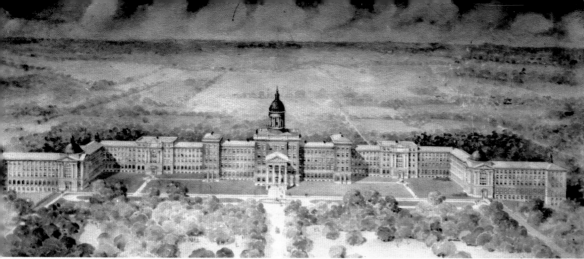

Building Project

By 1907 the building designed for no more than three hundred patients held more than six hundred. City officials finally committed to a building plan to relieve the situation. The design called for four additional wings to be added on either side of the existing hospital. A "maniacal building" for especially difficult or dangerous cases would also be built as a freestanding structure on the back grounds. The new construction would provide room for two thousand patients and three hundred staff.

Excavation began on October 6, 1907. By October 6, 1910, the additions to the west wing were complete. On October 24, the female patients that were staying at the poor house were transferred to their new accommodations. On November 28, those that had been housed at State Hospital No. 3 in the town of Nevada made the trip home to St. Louis.

The east wing was finished by January of 1911. During February of that year, the male patients from the poor house returned, as well as those that had been staying at State Hospital No. 4 in Farmington.

Along with the new buildings came a new name. St. Louis City Insane Asylum would now be known as City Sanitarium. By March 31, 1911, the sanitarium's census was 1,814.

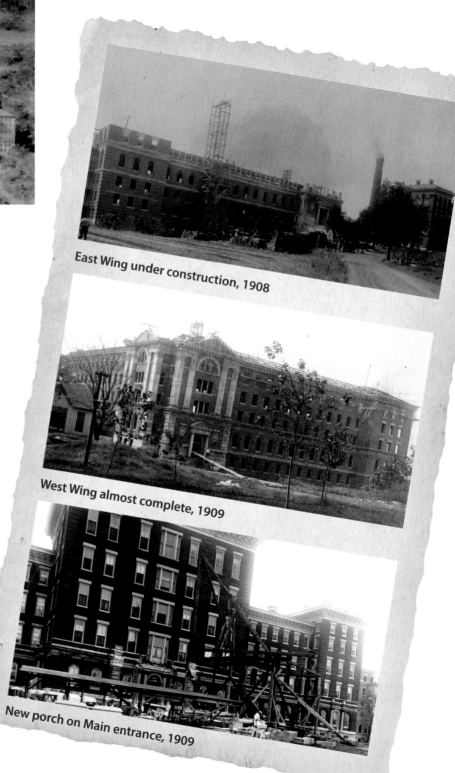

East Wing under construction, 1908

West Wing almost complete, 1909

New porch on Main entrance, 1909

New Building Materials

Even though city officials had balked and grumbled for years regarding the funding of the building project, a surprising amount of care was put into choosing the materials and finishes for the final product. Each entrance of the new wings was flanked with granite pillars, two cartouches topped with lion heads, and terra cotta carvings. White English veined marble wainscoting with light gray Tennessee marble bases lined the interior staircases. Terrazzo flooring in complementary colors was chosen for its hygienic and aesthetic properties. The wards themselves were built with high ceilings, large windows, and marble-lined bathrooms. The walls were painted in light colors such as mint and peach for their calming influence.

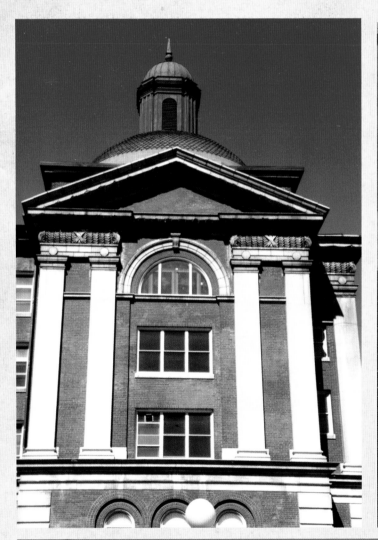
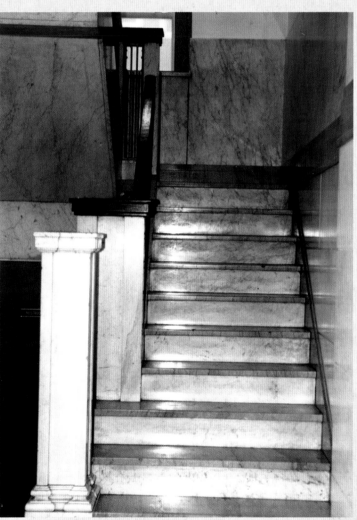
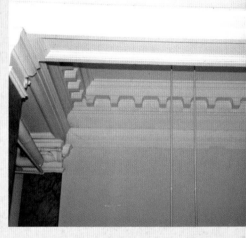
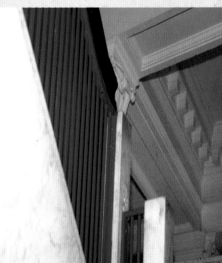

Ideal Qualities in Staff

The nature of the work in the asylum called for a special set of skills. According to Dr. Howard, the ideal attendant "must be courageous, firm, patient, forbearing, intelligent, and sympathetic." Most attendants lived on the wards with their charges and therefore had to be willing to sacrifice a "normal" family life. In addition, attendants were expected to assist with medical interventions, break up fights, and keep their patients clean. All of this was to be done, in 1881, for ninety-three cents a day. While that number would certainly rise over the years, the attendants would remain the lowest paid of all hospital employees.

Due to the low pay and sometimes onerous duties, resignations and discharges took place on a daily basis.

JUST A FEW EXAMPLES FROM THE 1920S WERE:

"Very sleepy headed."

"Querulous disposition."

"She seemed a very stubborn person."

"Habitually absented himself from duty, without permission to do so."

"She was hysterical for days."

"Borrowed money from a patient and did not return it."

"Frequenting places were intoxicating liquor is served."

"Interfering with married couples' affairs."

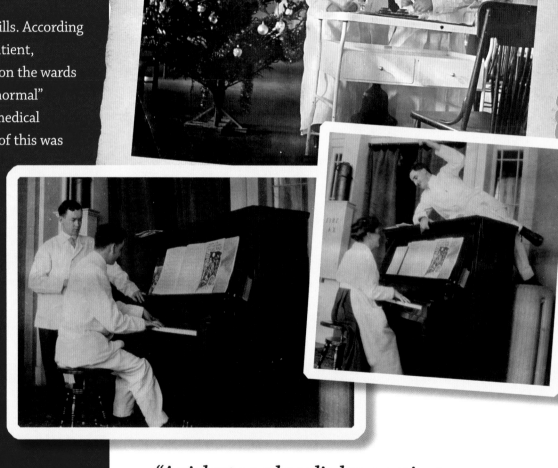

"A violent word applied to a patient was followed by immediate dismissal of the offender, for I hold that an uncontrollable tongue presupposes the existence of uncontrollable fists." —Dr. Runge, 1896

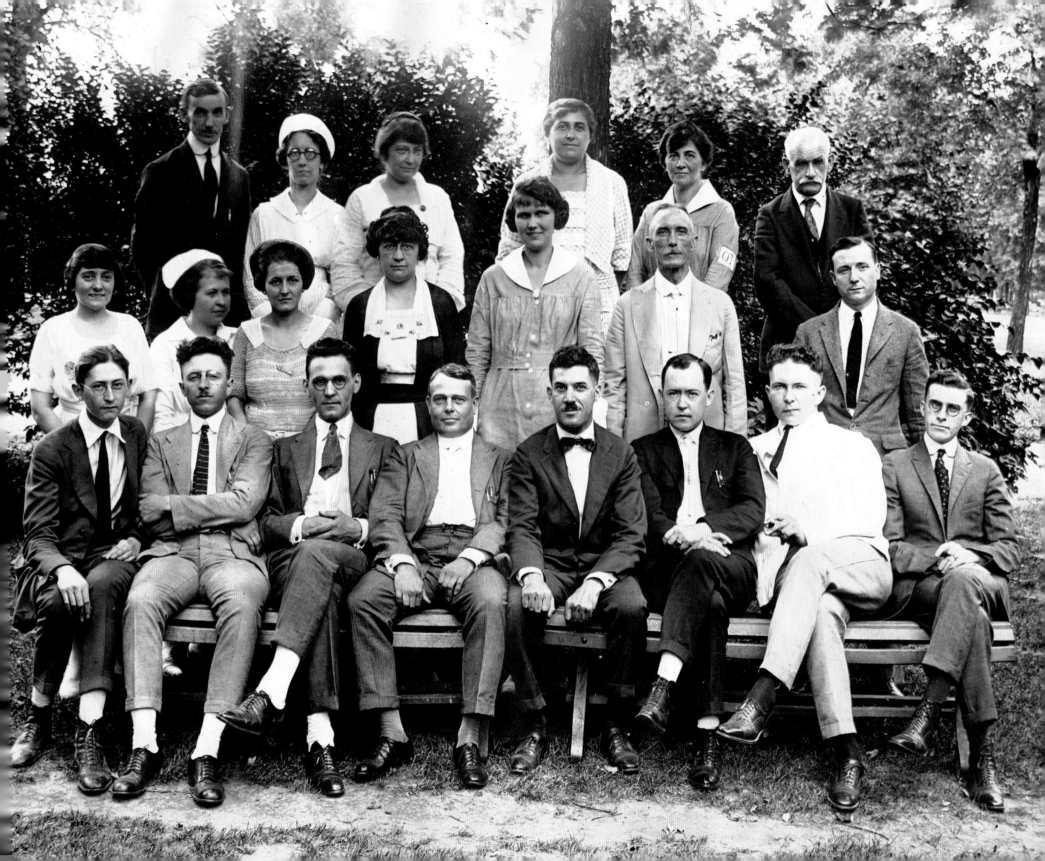

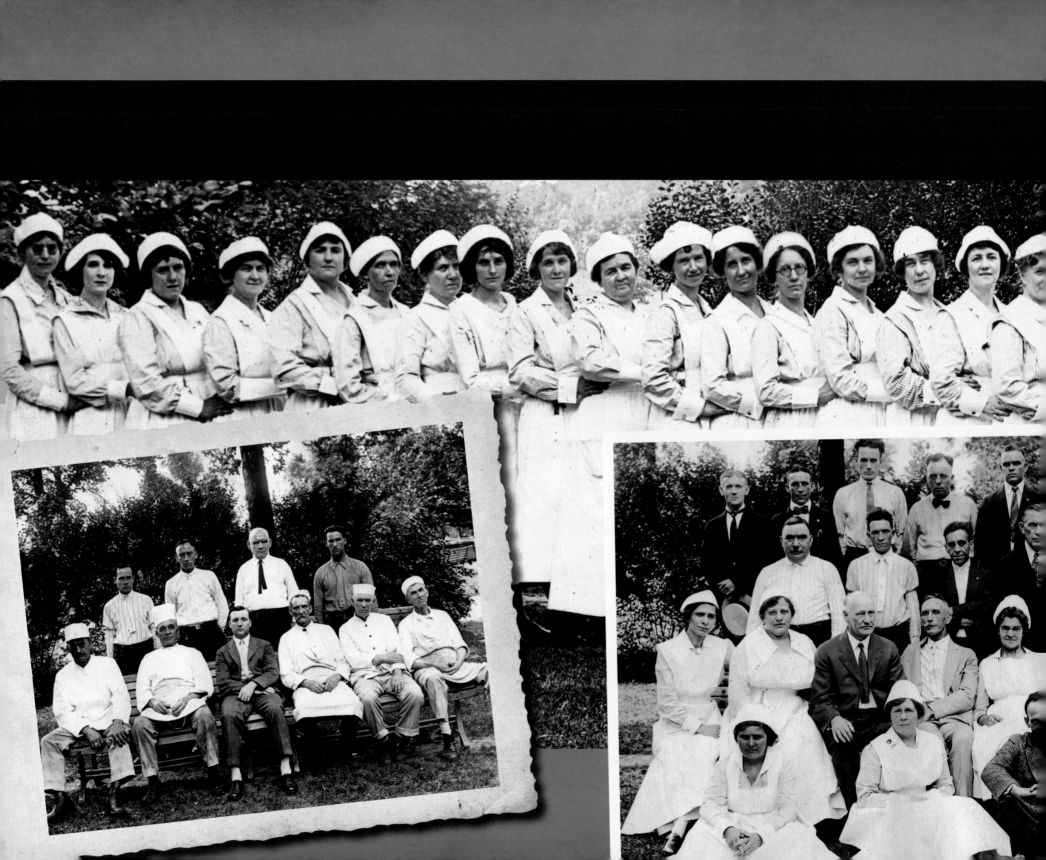

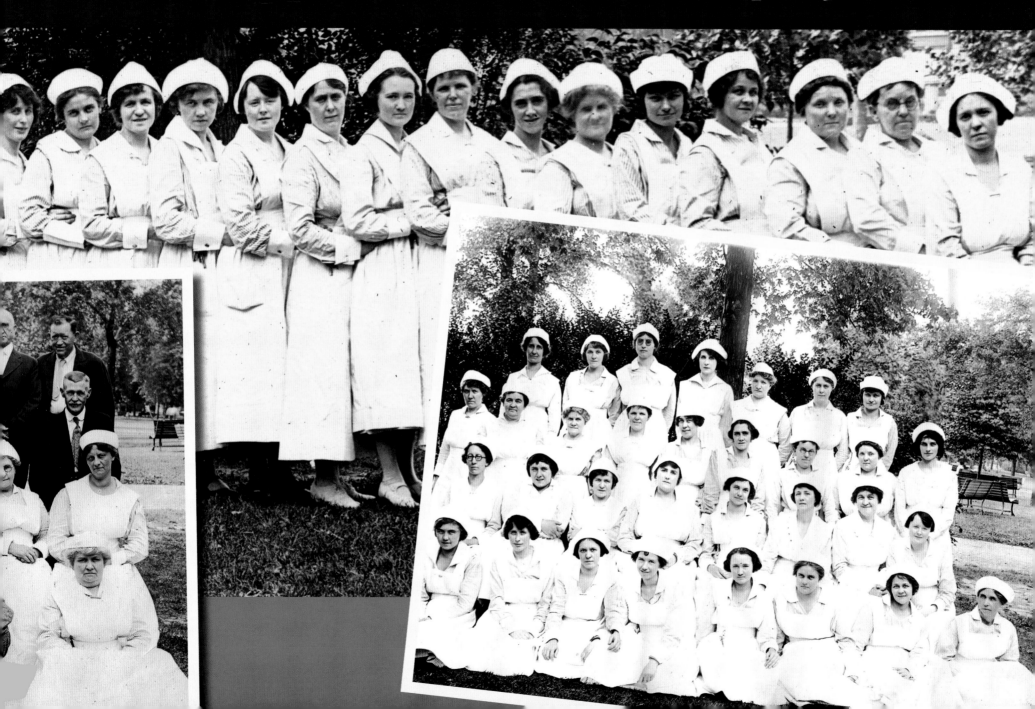

City Sanitarium Employees

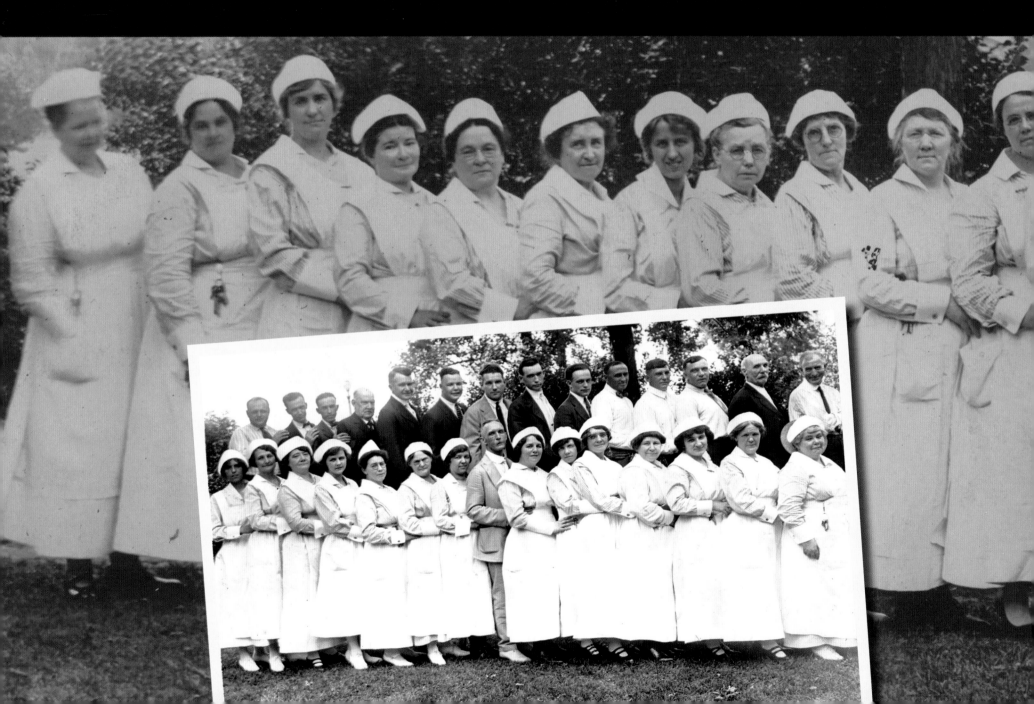

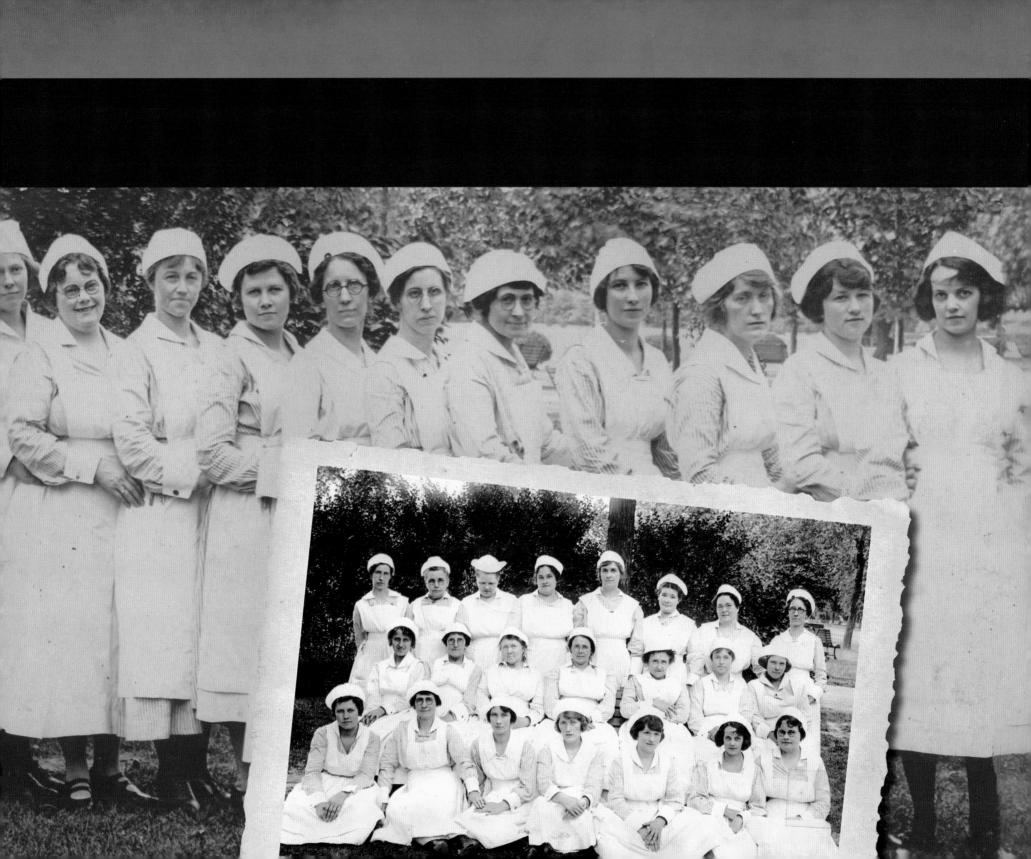

Annals of City San

In 1914 Dr. Johns was approached by the Committee on the History of the Institutional Care of the Insane in the United States and Canada regarding the history of the sanitarium. Longtime employee Robert E. Lee Gibson eagerly accepted the assignment and began work on what would become one of the most valuable sources of historical information on the institution, *The Annals of the City Sanitarium*. Gibson was hired as an assistant clerk to the steward in 1890. In addition to his organizational skills, he was known in St. Louis literary circles as an author and poet. His eye for detail and personable writing style made the annals accessible as well as informative. The work documented the first fifty years of the hospital and included anecdotes, descriptions of buildings, statistics on numerous topics, and even a poem "submitted" by an old staircase.

The Annals was thought lost from around 1920 until 1940, when it turned up among papers in a file room. Fortunately, the superintendent at the time, Dr. Grogan, recognized its value and had it preserved.

Annals

of the

City Sanitarium

Compiled under the Direction

of the Superintendent

at the

City of St. Louis, Missouri

In the Month of March in the Year of Our Lord

1915

to

His Honor, The Mayor

This Little Volume

The Annals of the City Sanitarium, St. Louis

is Respectfully Dedicated

This volume, Annals of the City Sanitarium, was copied from a manuscript found among a number of books and papers in the file room of the Sanitarium. The manuscript was unsigned but I am informed it was compiled and written in 1915 by Mr. Robert E. Lee Gibson, a man of reputation as a poet and writer, who then held the position of Steward of the Sanitarium.

The Annals begin with a resolution dated December 10, 1863, presented by Judge H. Fisse of the St. Louis County Court, proposing the erection of the "St. Louis County Insane Asylum". There follows an account of the laying of the corner stone which event took place, December 2, 1864. The original buildings and several additions are described in some detail and reference is made to difficulties encountered during the progress of the construction.

The Annals include a great amount of statistical data: the number of patients present, admissions, deaths, discharges and maintenance costs. The names of the Superintendents and other officials are set forth and brief summaries are given of some of the annual reports. The Annals record events of historical importance and relate many incidents of human interest.

The Annals close with excerpts from the Annual Report of the Superintendent, Doctor George A. Johns, March 31, 1914.

F. M. Grogan, M.D.,
Superintendent

Copied
April
1940

Treatment Focus: Occupational Therapy

Occupational therapy, as its name implies, was designed to keep patients occupied and engaged. Creative and entertaining activities had been around from the beginning; however, in 1918 a formal occupational therapy department was established. Trained occupational therapists from Washington University were employed to assess patients' fitness, interests, and skills. The therapists wasted no time in designing tailored programs to keep patients busy while benefiting the hospital.

Soon various shops specializing in specific activities were spread throughout the sanitarium. Male patients tended to be placed in pursuits such as carpentry, grounds maintenance, shoe repair, and bookbinding, while female patients worked in the sewing room and helped in the kitchen. By the mid-1920s, community interest and involvement in the hospital led to occupational therapy bazaars. The craft fairs of their day, the bazaars featured items made exclusively by the patients for sale to friends, relatives, and the public. Baskets, wooden toys, felted flowers, and more were available. Funds raised went back into the department to purchase materials as well as provide entertainments.

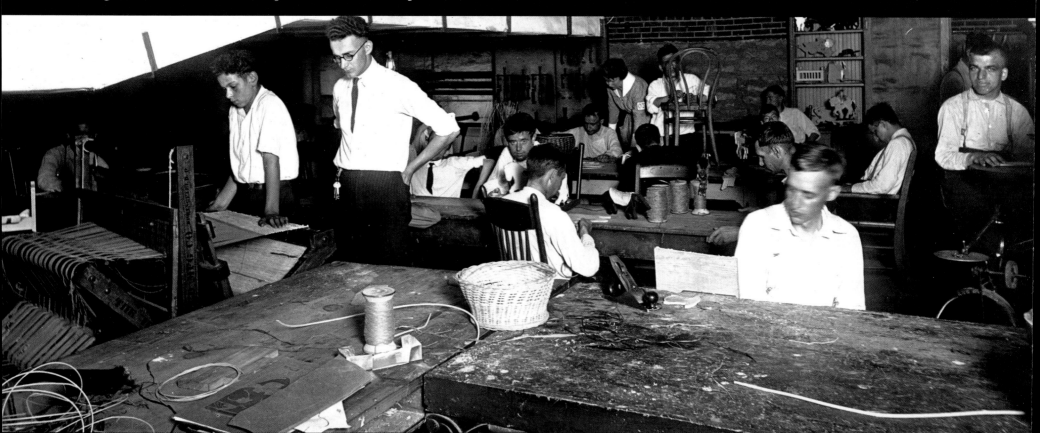

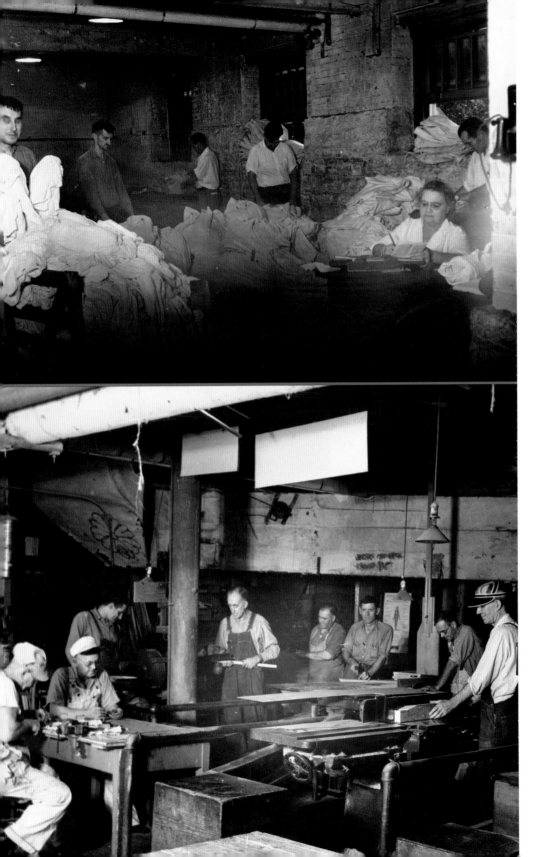

"*Absence of mental food must invariably lead to mental scurvy and starvation, and we have no more right to starve the brain than the stomach.*"

—Dr. Runge, 1903

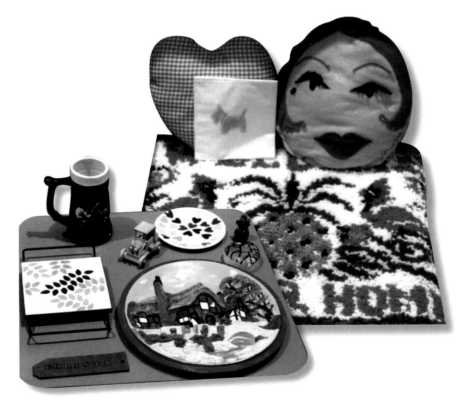

City Sanitarium in War Time

The management of an underfunded and overcrowded institution was a challenge during peace time. Only the patriotic sense of duty to persevere from both staff and patients could get the sanitarium through World War I. Population at this point was hovering around 2,300, while male staff members were leaving in droves to join the military. Attendant staff were hit the hardest; however, workers from all major departments, including physicians went off to fight.

During the war years, Superintendent Johns relied on female staff, patient cooperation, and sheer grit to manage. The majority of produce came from the garden, and it was not uncommon to go without meat in order to save money. Meanwhile, Red Cross volunteers and occupational therapists kept patients busy knitting to help the troops. In 1917, eighty-eight patients (eight men and eighty women) produced 246 sweaters, 34 helmet liners, and 96 scarves for the boys overseas.

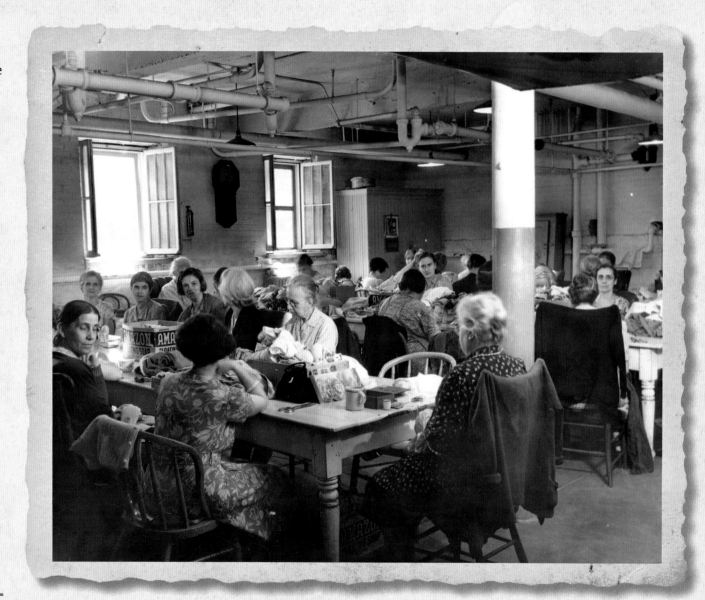

Sewing Room in southeast basement, 1920

Special School No. 2 at City Sanitarium

It was not unusual for children to be admitted to the sanitarium. Psychiatric help for youth simply did not exist, and the School for the Feeble Minded experienced the same overcrowded conditions as the hospital on Arsenal. Superintendents long expressed concern regarding youth intermingled with adult patients and tried to segregate younger patients accordingly.

In 1921 a partnership was formed between the sanitarium and the St. Louis Public School system. The hospital agreed to fund the construction of a small school house if the school district would provide teachers. Special School No. 2 at City Sanitarium opened its doors to a class of thirty-one pupils. Ms. Nellie Bashaw and Ms. Pauline Lopheimer, educators, described the children as ranging from "6–18 years of age with a mental age of 3–8." The school day began with exercise, followed by lessons in reading and simple arithmetic. Practical skills such as grooming, presentation, and deportment were also included. By the end of the first year the school program was considered a success, with an attendance rate of nearly 97 percent. A setback occurred in 1922 when a pupil attempted to burn the building to the ground. Fortunately, only half of the building was lost in the blaze, and classes continued in the main building while it was rebuilt.

The school building would remain on campus as a storage area until 1971 when it was, ironically, burned to the ground by another disgruntled patient.

Dr. Raeder and baby born at City San, 1914

Breathing Room

The patient population continued to grow during the 1920s and, as before, it took several years of nagging before the city decided to act. In 1925 approval was given for an expansion, and after two years of construction, the Employees' Building was ready to provide relief. The three-story, three-wing building was located on the corner of the property at Arsenal and Brannon. It provided room for more than three hundred attendants and physicians, freeing up considerable room inside the main building. For the first time in a decade, patients no longer had to set up cots in the hallways. Unfortunately, this freedom would only last for a few years before the cot situation became necessary once again.

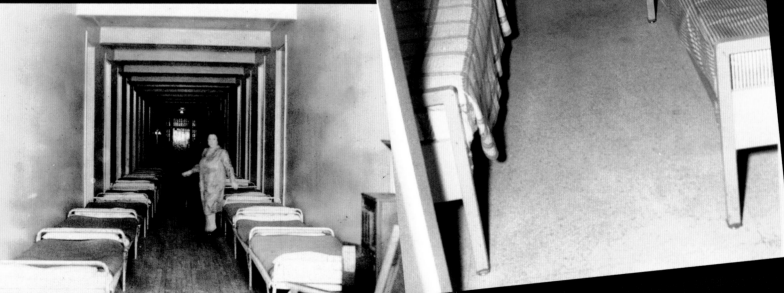

Cots in hallways for extra sleeping areas, 1932

Three person bedroom, 1940s

Right: **Nurses and Employees' Building, 1930**

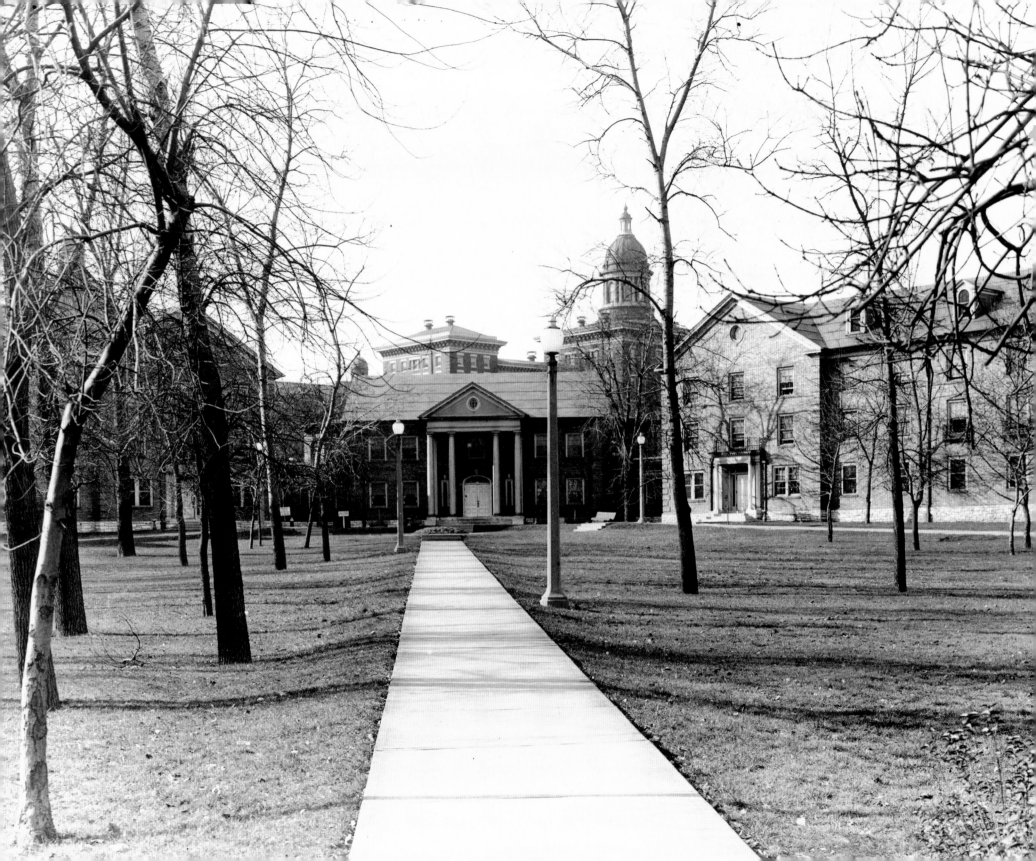

A Splendid Auditorium

Included in the 1925 Employees' Building plan were funds for the construction of, in the words of Superintendent Lee, a "splendid auditorium, gymnasium, and dining room." The two-story addition replaced the rear piazzas on the first four floors of the center building. The gymnasium was fitted with the best hardwood floors, large windows, and an upper balcony. At the rear of the area was a complete stage, including two dressing rooms, lighting, and curtains. Including the seating in the balcony, the entire area could accommodate over one thousand audience members for a variety of entertainments. Thanks to the generous donations of benefactors, a "Powers Motion Picture Machine of the very best kind" was installed for weekly viewing parties.

Beneath the gymnasium and auditorium was a bright and airy dining room and kitchen. The new space allowed employees the opportunity to enjoy hot meals and conversation throughout the day. This freedom was much appreciated by those that spent long hours isolated on wards throughout the grounds.

1925

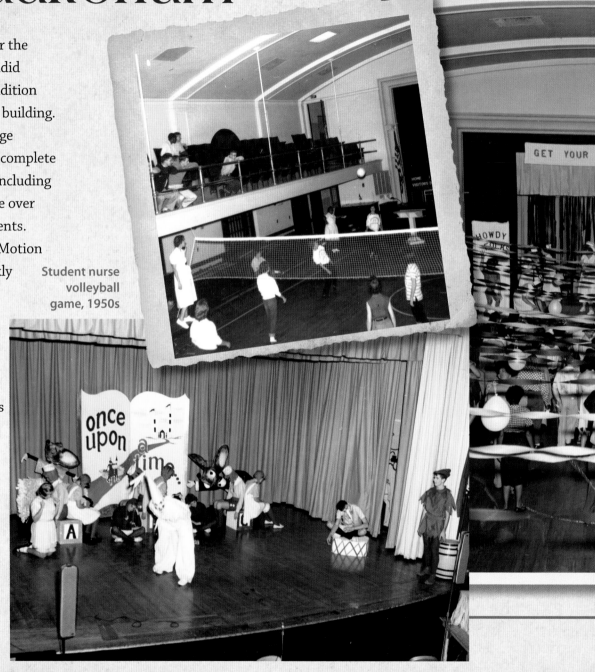

Student nurse volleyball game, 1950s

Performance of *Once Upon a Time,* 1950s

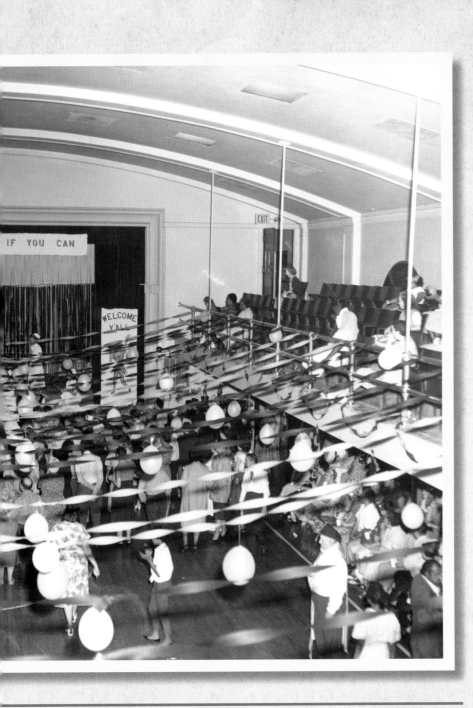

Sadie Hawkins Halloween Dance, 1961

The Trials and Tribulations of Dr. Lee

In 1925 a young, politically minded doctor was appointed superintendent by the newly elected mayor, Victor Miller. Dr. E. J. Lee Jr. immediately cleaned house by firing or harassing employees that did not support Miller's election. While morally questionable at best and illegal at worst, his connections with the mayor's office did result in funding for much-needed construction. Eventually Lee was promoted to the Health Commissioner's office, but would get his own comeuppance with the election of Bernard Dickmann. Lee found himself out of a job and out of luck. He remained in St. Louis and heckled politicians and the City Sanitarium via editorials in the local newspapers.

Treatment Focus: Vocational Rehabilitation

Therapeutic work, or vocational rehabilitation, was used from the beginning of the asylum's history to assist in patient recovery as well as make up for staffing shortages. Originally built in the "country," the hospital was intended to supply at least some of its own food via gardening. Well into the 1940s, patients could be found tending to a variety of vegetable plants on the back lawns.

Patient workers were assisted in these endeavors by the asylum's team of mules. The mules helped with farm work, hauling, and grounds maintenance. Each day a group of patient workers would hitch the mules to carts and drive the perimeter of the hospital's land, picking up trash and tending to the grounds.

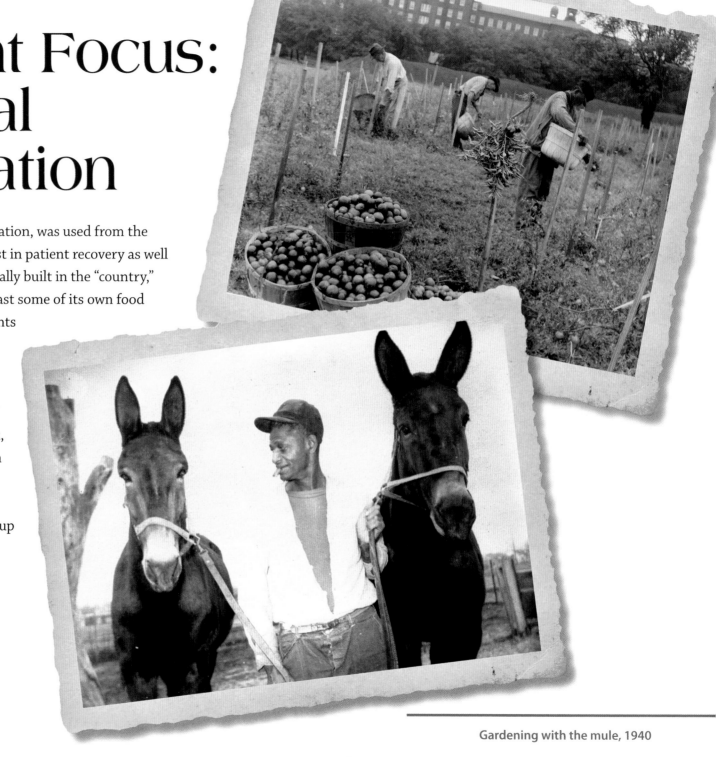

Gardening with the mule, 1940

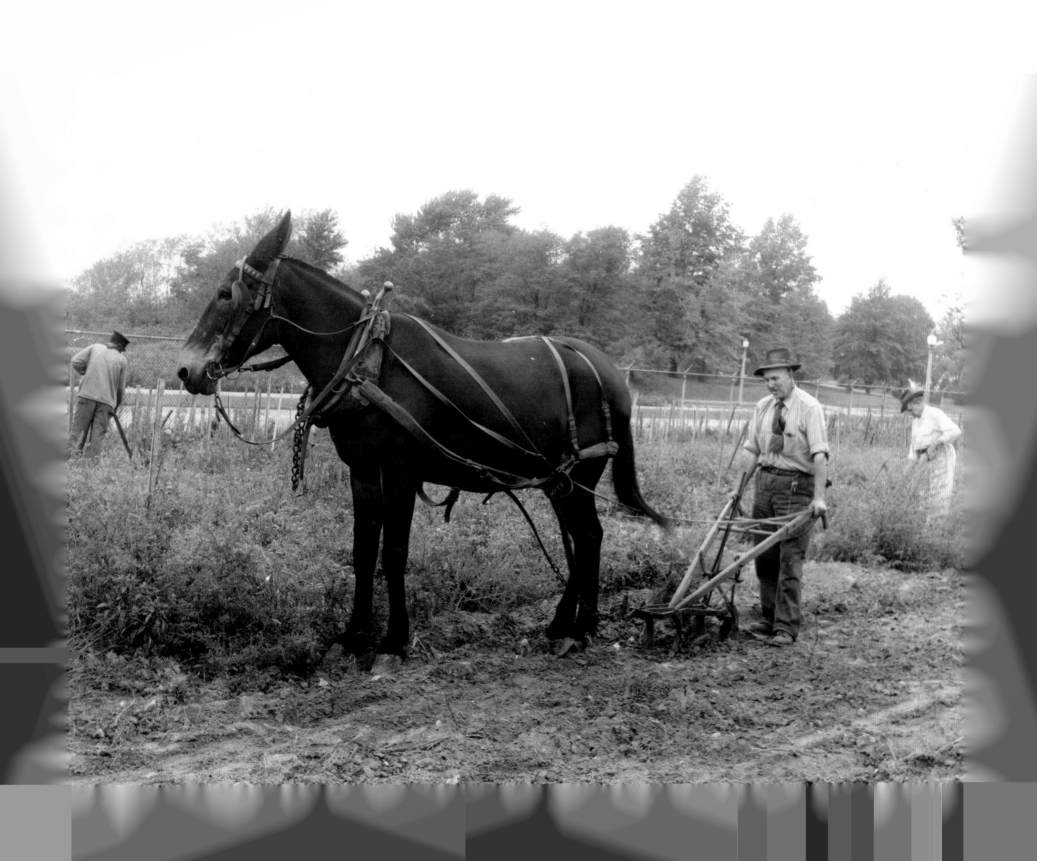

Dr. Louis H. Kohler

Louis Hirsch Kohler was born and raised in New Castle, Pennsylvania. He enlisted as a private in World War I and, upon his return, attended medical school at St. Louis University. After graduating in 1924, Dr. Kohler served internships at both City Hospital and City Sanitarium. Fascinated with the workings of the mind, he decided to focus his career on helping those with mental illness. In 1925 he accepted a resident physician position at the sanitarium. Within two years, he had been promoted to assistant superintendent. His work focused on the admissions unit, where he specialized in early interventions in an effort to minimize long-term hospitalization. He encouraged the use of treatments such as hydrotherapy and occupational therapy over restraints and isolation. He insisted that treatment could not be successful unless a proper rapport was built between doctor and patient. To this end, he prided himself on knowing the names of all his charges as well as the majority of the other patients.

In 1941, following the transfer of Dr. Grogan to the health department, he was named superintendent. His plans for improving sanitarium care were interrupted by World War II, when alumni from St. Louis University formed the 70th General Army Hospital. Committed to his country, Dr. Kohler took a leave of absence and went off to fight.

Upon returning in 1946, he picked up where he had left off. Over the next decade, he instituted programs and policies that would revolutionize both the hospital and the practice of mental health care itself. The relationships he fostered with local universities ensured that his patients would have access to high-quality care and provided students with hands-on learning opportunities. His commitment to making mental health care accessible without long-term hospitalization led to the establishment of the community health care model.

Despite all of his accomplishments, Dr. Kohler preferred to keep a quiet profile. He never married and instead spent most of his time among his patients and staff. He was always available to lend a listening ear and encouraging word. Upon his retirement in 1964, he asked for no parties or accolades and instead spent time fishing and relaxing. After his passing in 1983, his estate was used to provide scholarships for St. Louis University medical students as well as to contribute to other charities.

"*We can become angry and resentful of God because of our illness or we can accept the lesson it gives us in learning new ways of adjusting.*"
—Dr. Kohler, 1961

Treatment Focus: Hydrotherapy

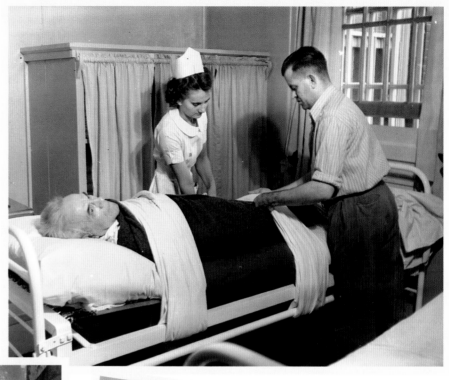

Prior to the development of psychotropic medications in the 1950s, hydrotherapy provided a relatively inexpensive yet effective treatment for patients. Various methods of hydrotherapy were used in mental health care throughout the country, but wet packs and continuous tub baths were the treatments of choice at City Sanitarium.

Wet packs consisted of swaddling a patient in wet sheets topped with a wool cover. The patient would remain wrapped until the sheets reached body temperature. Continuous tub baths involved the patient relaxing in a large bathtub. A tight canvas cover stretched over the top of the tub and around the patient's neck, allowing the temperature of the water to remain steady. In each method, the duration of treatment and temperature of the water depended upon the patient's diagnosis. Cold water was thought to help those experiencing mania, while warm water helped invigorate those with melancholy. Both treatments were provided in specially designed rooms located at the end of the wards to promote quiet and relaxation.

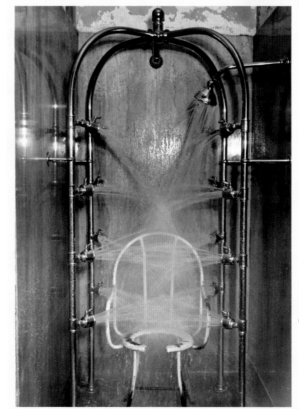

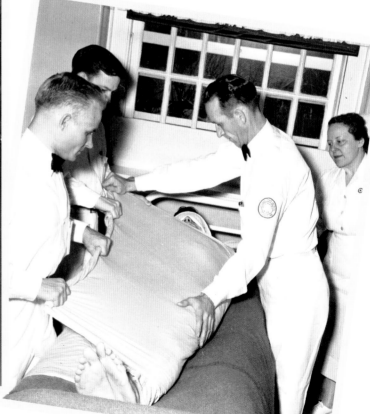

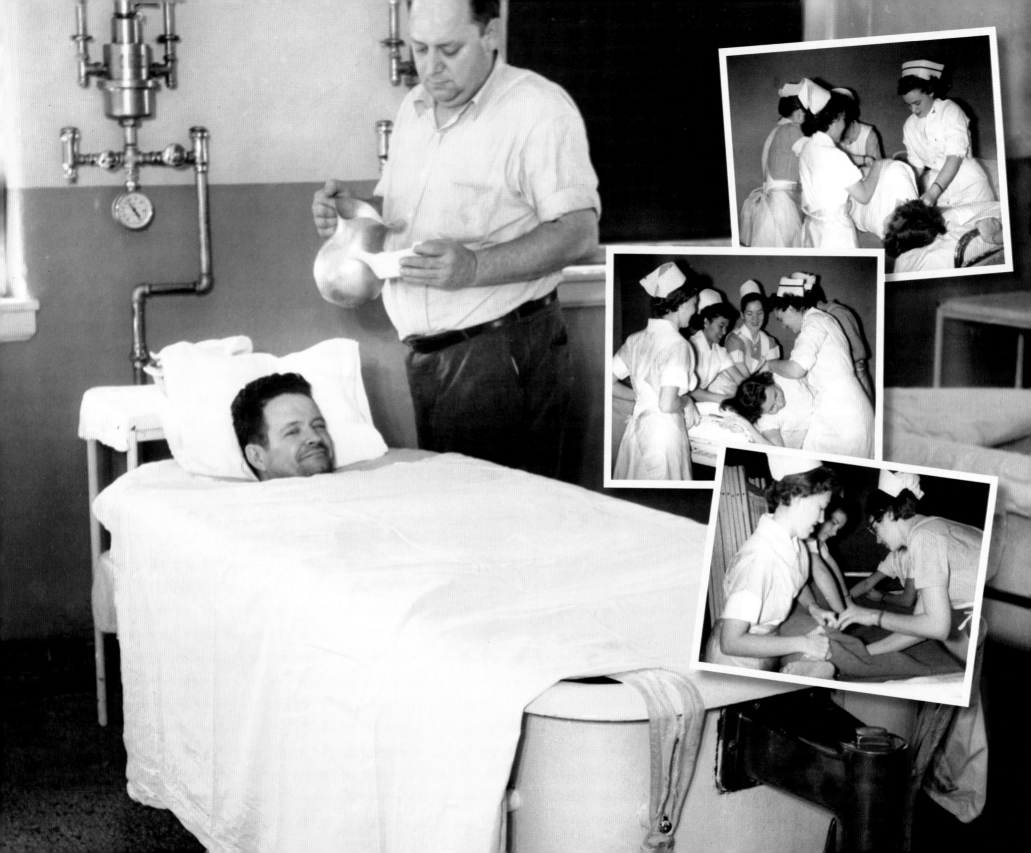

New Deal Workers

While the rest of the country struggled, City Sanitarium found itself benefiting during the Great Depression. For the first time, there was a surplus of applicants to choose from as well as affordable labor through the New Deal. In particular, the Public Works Administration (PWA) assisted with several long-overdue construction projects. The outside of the building was cleaned from top to bottom for the first time in its history. A solarium was added to the end of each hall, providing occupants with large windows and much-needed space. Unfortunately, while the PWA workers were enthusiastic, they were not all equally skilled. Tales of workers sliding off the roof, getting tangled in harnesses, and needing to be rescued off the water tower were common. That said, by the end of the 1930s the sanitarium had gotten a facelift and the patients had stories to share.

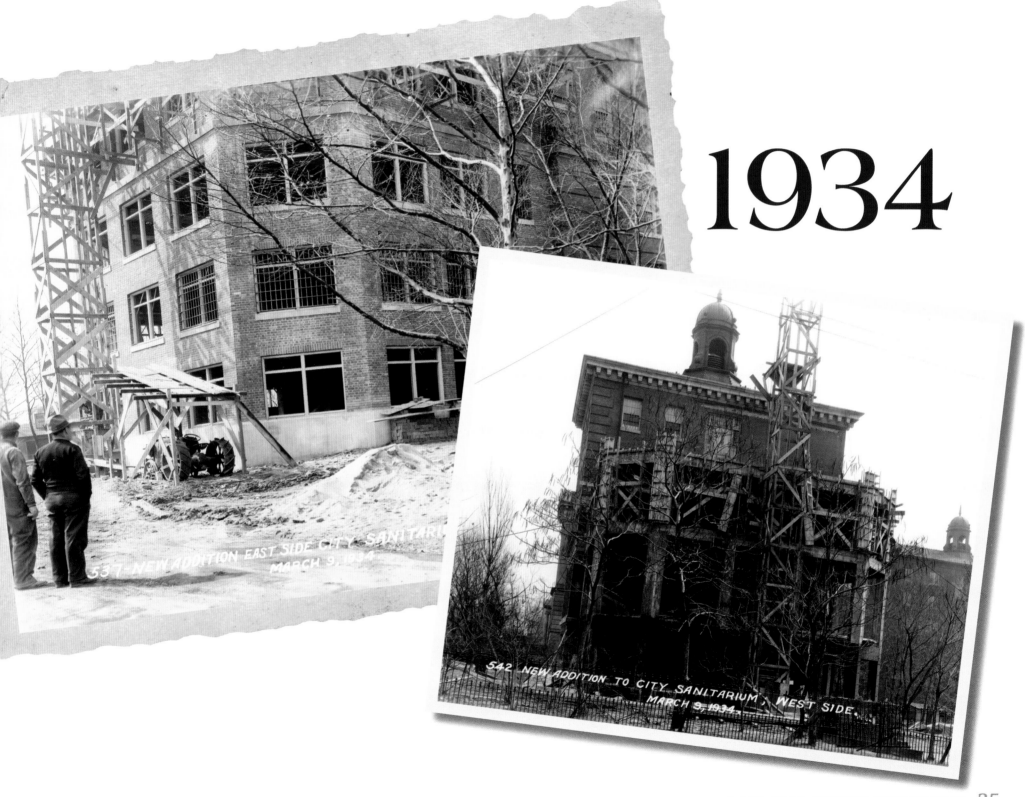

1934

537 - NEW ADDITION EAST SIDE CITY SANITARIUM
MARCH 9, 1934

542 NEW ADDITION TO CITY SANITARIUM, WEST SIDE
MARCH 9, 1934

Treatment Focus: Shocks to the System

In addition to lobotomy and hydrotherapy, several new treatments were developed to literally shock the patient back to health. Lacking any formal direction or guidelines from governing bodies such as the American Medical Association, psychiatrists began utilizing these methods on their patients.

Theelin, or estrone, therapy involved giving female patients experiencing hysteria and psychosis large doses of estrogen hormones.

Deep radiotherapy consisted of prolonged exposure to radiation under specially designed x-ray machines. Individuals with end-stage syphilis were given malarial treatment to flush out toxins. The goal of insulin therapy was to induce a coma by dosing patients with high levels of insulin. Metrazol therapy involved the direct injection of Metrazol (pentamethylenetetrazol) into the blood stream. The resulting two- to three-minute seizures were thought to restart the brain. Finally, there was electric shock therapy, in which a patient was held down by a squad of nurses and attendants while the doctor applied shocks through electrodes held to the patient's head.

All of the above treatments, with the exception of electric shock, were eventually found to be either ineffective or downright dangerous and fell out of use.

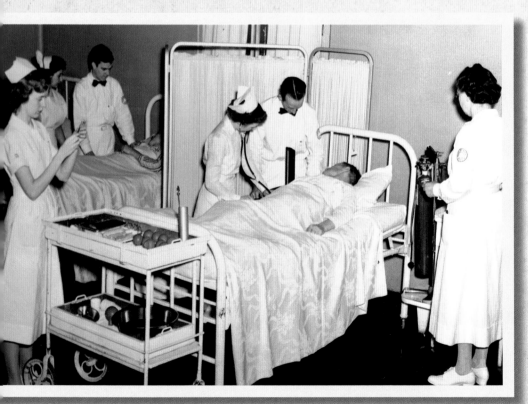

Dr. Grundel and student nurses, 1940s

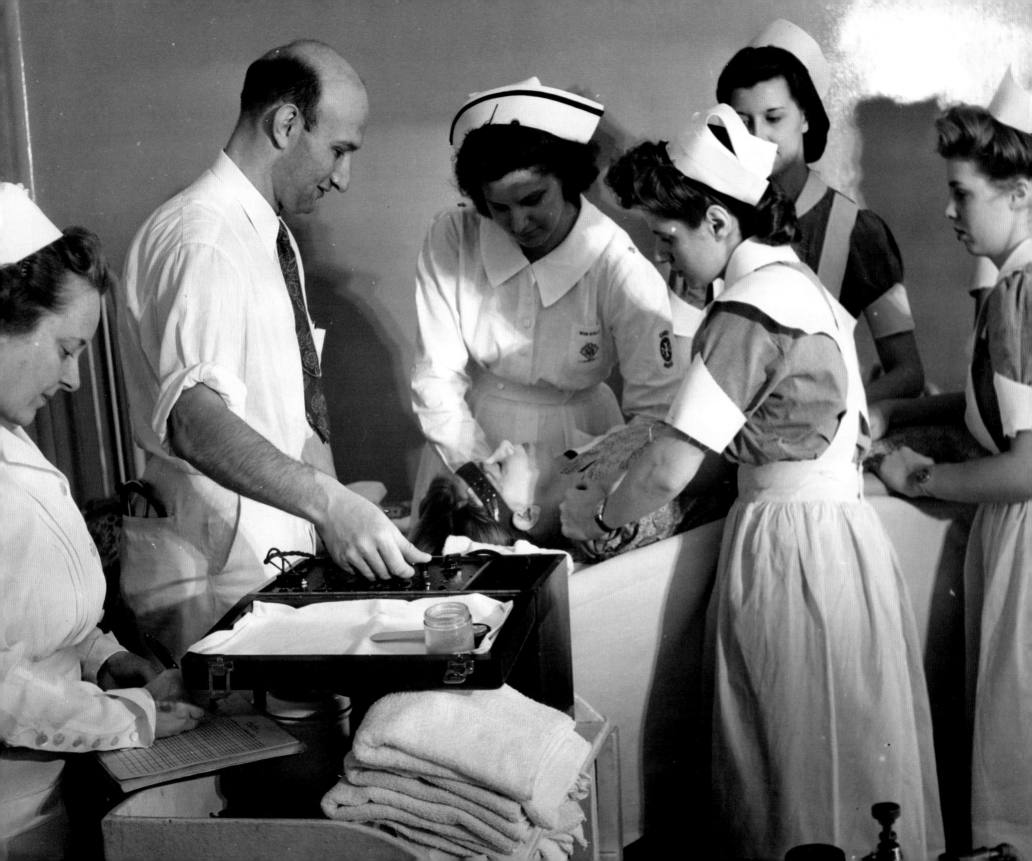

Student Nurse Affiliation 1935

Prior to the 1930s it was not uncommon for state hospitals and asylums to be staffed by attendants and physicians only. Trained nursing was a developing field and tended to focus on physical rather than mental needs.

As more trained nurses entered practice and asylum populations continued to grow, it seemed time to introduce a course specifically on psychiatric care. In 1933, members of the Missouri State Nurses' Association and the Missouri State League of Nursing Education began work on developing a psychiatric course for nursing students. Delegates from both organizations toured the five public psychiatric hospitals in Missouri to determine which one would provide the best learning experience.

Factors considered included the attitude of administration towards nurses, location of the hospital, and the facilities available. State Hospital No. 3 in Nevada, Missouri, was quickly eliminated after the superintendent expressed his opinion that trained nurses were "supercilious." State Hospitals No. 1 in Fulton and No. 2 in St. Joseph were considered too far from major cities. State Hospital No. 4 in Farmington was lovely; sadly, it could provide no housing for nursing students.

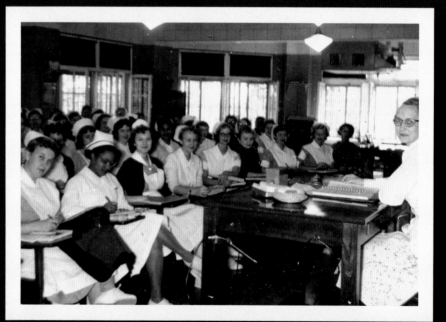

City Sanitarium, on the other hand, met all of their needs. It was conveniently located by several nursing schools and was a stop on the major public transportation routes. The large Employees' Building provided housing, dining, and entertainment facilities. Finally, sanitarium administration saw the value in education and the opportunity to utilize students for staffing purposes.

Nursing educators Augusta Bigler, Dillie Gulmi, and Mabel Leavitt were recruited from Cleveland, Ohio. Working with hospital administrators and city officials, the trio designed a six-month post-graduate curriculum. Everything was set to go when the city ran into its usual funding troubles. Eventually a compromise was reached in which City Sanitarium could provide room and board for the students if the Missouri nursing organizations covered the educators' salaries.

On April 1, 1935, classes began. The first group consisted of recently graduated nurses from St. Mary's, St. Luke's, City Hospital No. 1, and City Hospital No. 2. It was considered quite progressive at the time to allow the candidate from City Hospital No. 2, an institution designed for "colored" people, to study alongside the other three white women. However, sanitarium officials never questioned it, believing that qualified students of any background were welcome.

The psychiatric nursing program was declared a success after its first year. The curriculum, instructors, and patients made the experience valuable to those in the nursing field. Before long, Miss Bigler and Miss Gulmi were overwhelmed with applications. In order to accommodate more students, the class was shortened to three months and was soon adapted to become the psychiatric rotation in nursing school programs.

The psychiatric nursing program offered by City Sanitarium provided a valuable experience that wasn't available elsewhere in the Midwest. At the end of the decade, schools in Springfield, Kansas City, Independence, and Columbia were sending their students to St. Louis. By 1950 schools in Oklahoma, South Dakota, Tennessee, and even Hawaii had all placed nursing students at the San to learn the ins and outs of psychiatric work.

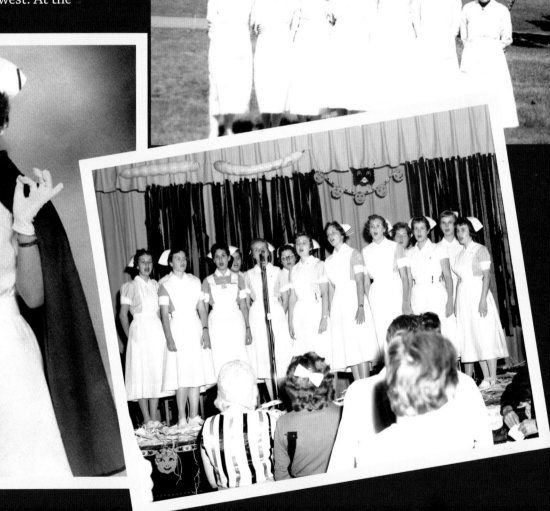

Dillie Rose Gulmi, RN

Registered nurse Dillie Rose Gulmi burst onto the City Sanitarium scene in 1935 when she agreed to accompany her friend Augusta Bigler to St. Louis in order to set up a psychiatric training program for student nurses. Always up for an adventure, she left her home in Cleveland and never looked back. Described as spunky, sassy, and energetic, Miss Gulmi epitomized the modern woman. She lived in her own house, drove her own car, and dedicated her career to the hospital. After Ms. Bigler retired, Miss Gulmi took her place as nursing educator and eventually rose through the ranks to become head of nursing and later assistant to the superintendent. Over the course of her time at St. Louis State Hospital, she was awarded with numerous commendations from civic and professional organizations. She retired after forty years of service but continued to be active with hospital staff and was a founding member of the Ole' Timers Club.

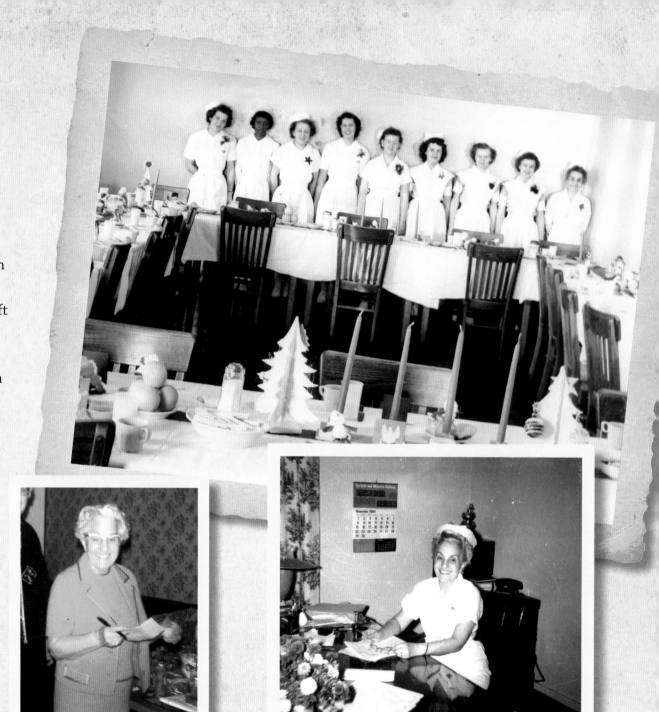

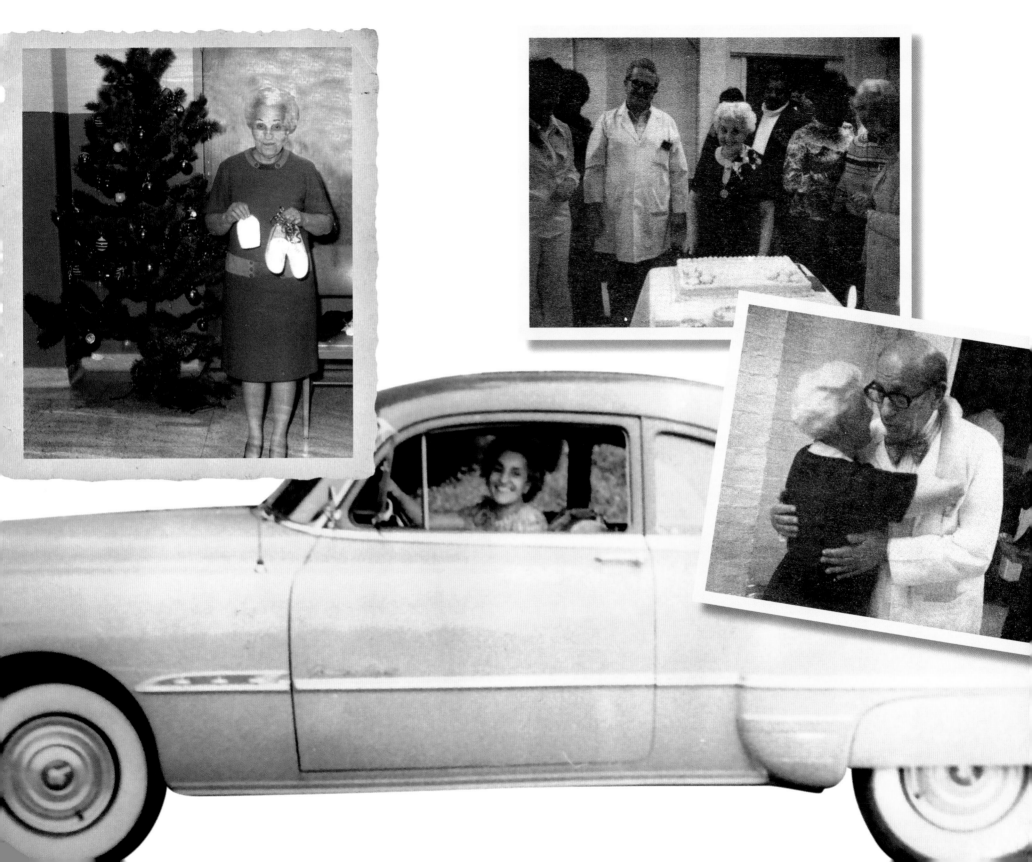

Student Nurses

During their time at the San, student nurses often found themselves away from home and faced with an intimidating environment. In order to boost morale, Miss Gulmi encouraged each class to form a student council to provide companionship and bonding opportunities. The classes from 1950 through 1967 took this a step farther by establishing various committees, including judicial, entertainment, and scrapbook.

The judicial committee ensured that students followed the rules of the sanitarium as well as those of their individual schools. For example, while on duty, students were expected to be in their complete school uniforms. The entertainment committee organized a faculty tea, wiener roast, and outings. The scrapbook committee documented everything in handmade albums. The scrapbooks provide insight into the daily lives of the nursing students as well as that of the hospital.

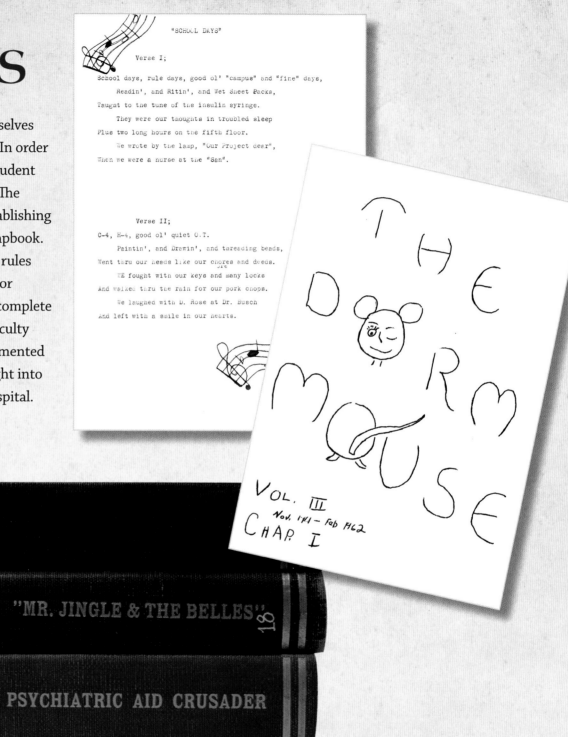

Student Nurse Scrapbooks

From 1950 to 1967, approximately seventy scrapbooks were made by student nurses. Each book had a unique title, class song, colors, and motto. An entire class photo was included, as well as a photo of the student council. Scrapbooks were as detailed and artistic as their individual creators. Some were irreverent, while others were almost overly dramatic. That said, all of the scrapbooks expressed gratitude toward the staff and care for the patients.

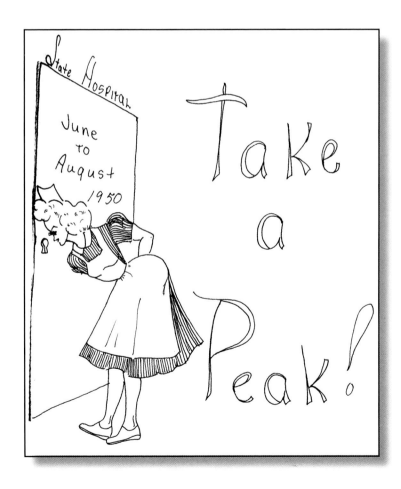

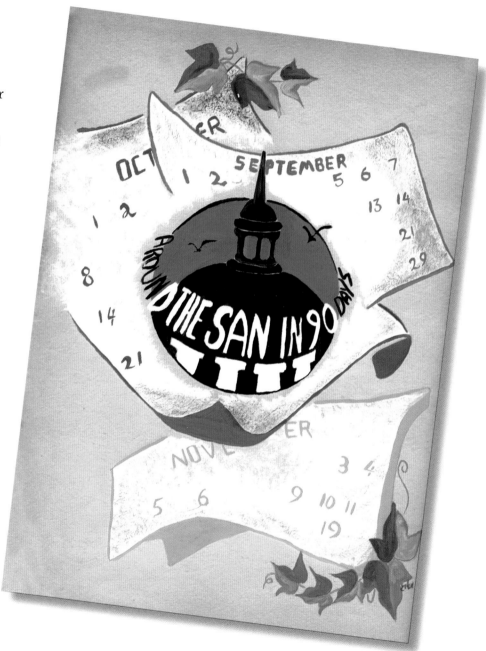

Dr. Leopold Hofstatter

Twinkle eyed and tongue in cheek, Dr. Hofstatter charmed nearly everyone he met with his stories and tall tales. The Austrian-born doctor came to the United States after being trained by some of the founding fathers of psychiatry. He settled in St. Louis and began an intensive search into the root causes of mental illness as well as possible cures. He and his colleagues brought groundbreaking, and controversial, treatments to City Sanitarium in an attempt to ease what he perceived as the suffering of his patients. He instructed countless numbers of student nurses and was described by more than one as "dreamy." Dr. Hofstatter served the Department of Mental Health in several leadership capacities, including as superintendent of St. Louis State Hospital in the late 1960s.

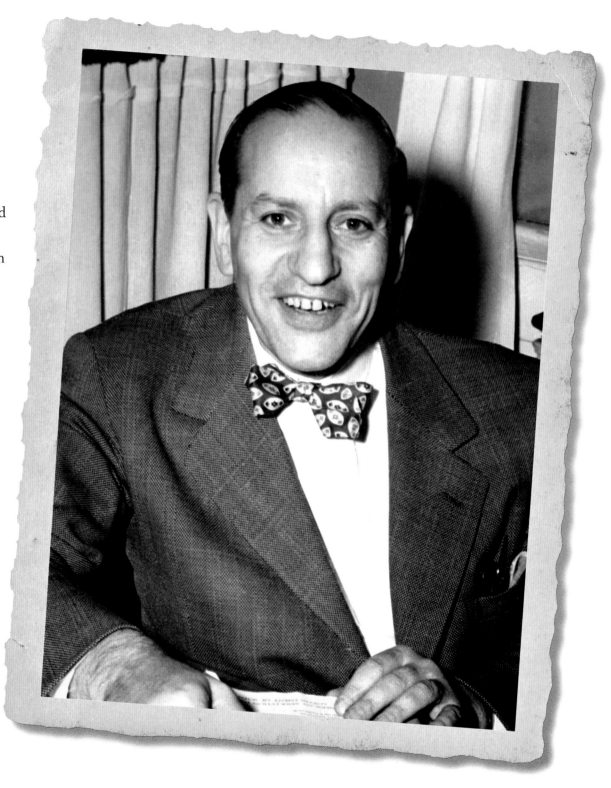

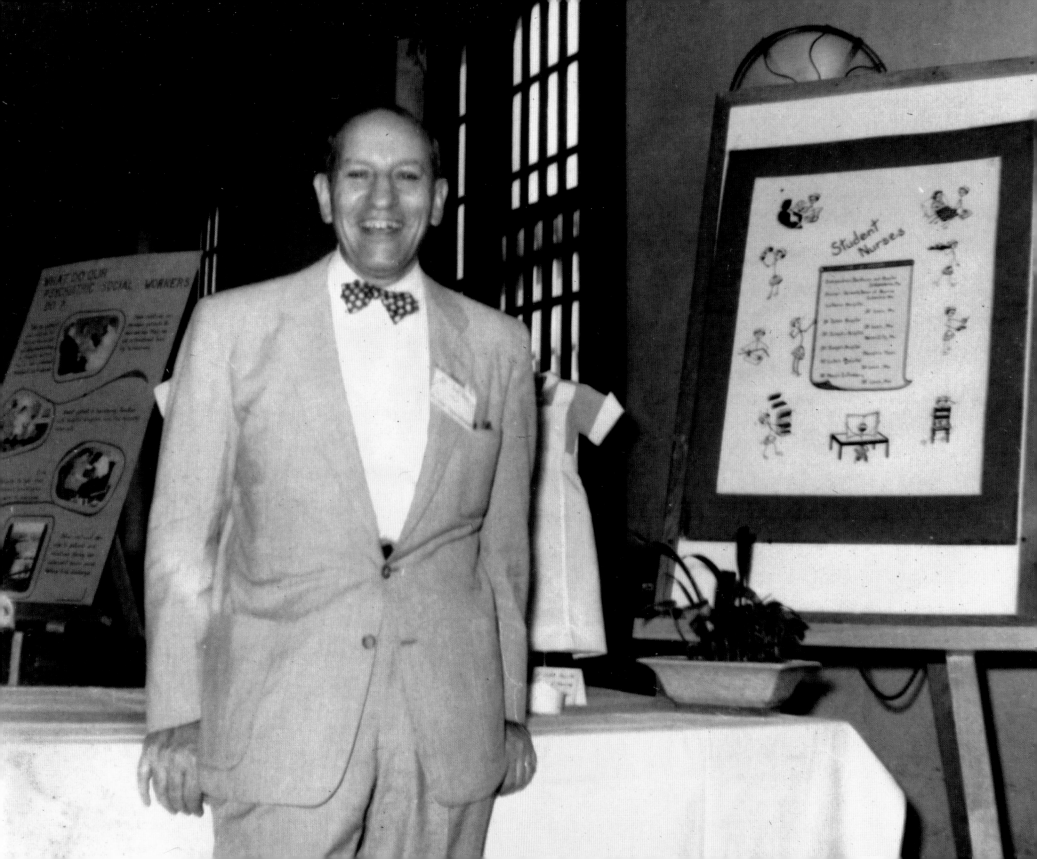

Treatment Focus: Psychosurgery

Outside the walls of City San, advances in psychiatry continued. In 1936 the prefrontal lobotomy was performed for the first time in the United States. This surgical procedure consisted of severing tissue in the brain's frontal lobes. Scientists speculated that the behaviors and beliefs of the mentally ill were rooted in this area and that disconnecting the tissues would cause the necessary personality shift to induce recovery.

By 1940 enough studies had been performed to satisfy City San's administration. The medical director, Dr. Anthony Busch, requested its inclusion into the treatments offered by the hospital. To develop the most effective method, Busch sought the assistance of Dr. Leopold Hofstatter from the neuropsychiatry department at Washington University. While the two examined cases from around the country, clinical staff began screening for patients to receive the operation.

Length and severity of illness as well as response to other forms of treatment such as hydrotherapy or electric shock were the main considerations. Less-well-defined measurements included excessive or inappropriate social behaviors that may or may not have been contrary to the social norms of the time.

In April 1941 Busch and Hofstatter began performing the procedure on patients. Unlike the lobotomies performed by Walter Freeman with a modified ice pick, those at City Sanitarium were conducted in the operating room with appropriate equipment. Following a "less is more" approach, the two doctors adapted the surgery in order to inflict the minimum amount of trauma to the brain.

By the mid-1950s the neurosurgery needs of the female population were overseen by Washington University surgeons, while St. Louis University surgeons assisted with male patients. A follow-up program was developed to help post-lobotomy patients adjust to their new lives. Despite these measures, the procedure was never proven to be a complete success. By the early 1960s it had been replaced by new psychiatric medications and talk therapies.

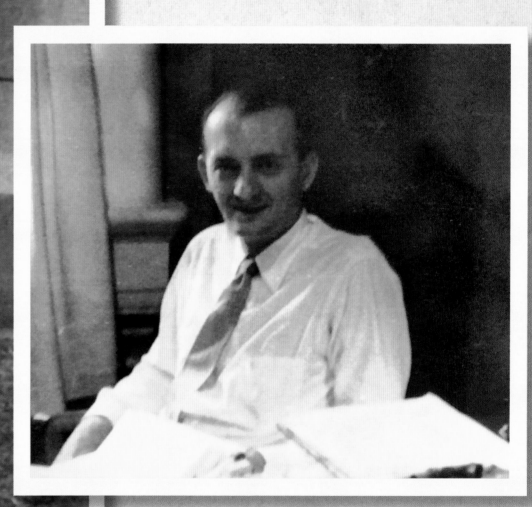

Dr. Leopold Hofstatter

Dr. Anthony Busch

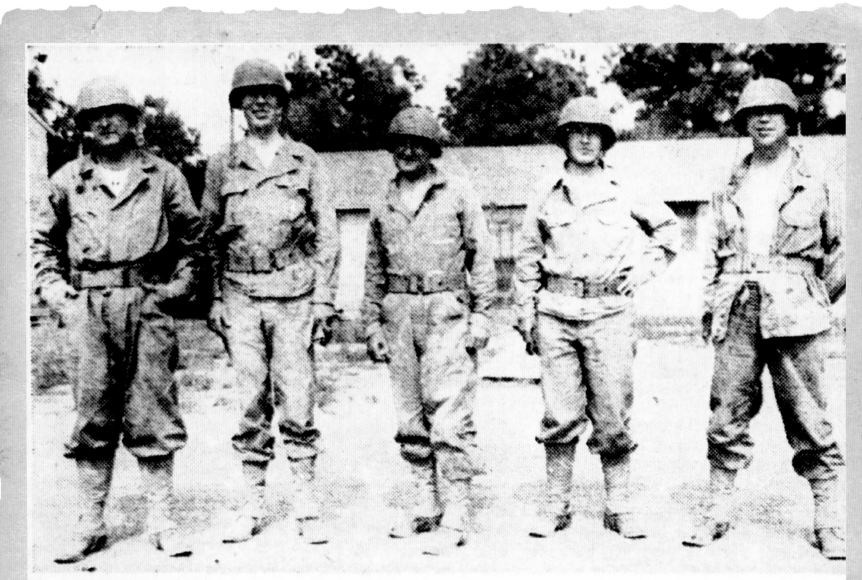

R, executive officer of St. Louis University's General Hospital Unit No. 70, on ı Italy. At right, a group of hospital officers. From left, WARRANT OFFICER RY B. CRIMMINS, chaplain, and LT. COL. LOUIS H. KOHLER, MAJ. RUT-DGE GISH and MAJ. S. HOOVER.

Dr. Kohler Goes to War (Again)

As its contribution to the war effort, the St. Louis University Medical School organized the 70th General Army Hospital. Graduates from across the area, several at the height of their careers, were asked to staff key positions. Among those called to serve were Dr. Curtis Lohr, superintendent of St. Louis County Hospital, and Father Harry Crimmins, president of the university itself. Despite the interruption to his own professional life, on May 6, 1943, Dr. Kohler joined as the chief of the Neuro-Psychiatry Unit as a major.

The 70th shipped out in August and was stationed for a year in North Africa. The medical staff treated heavy casualties, often working forty-eight hours at a stretch and dealing with supply shortages. When necessary, the doctors would give their own blood and plasma to help the wounded. After North Africa, the hospital spent the remainder of the war in Italy. To keep their spirits up, they listened to radio broadcasts, had a company orchestra, and shared letters from home.

By the end of the war, the hospital unit had earned multiple awards for excellence, and Dr. Kohler was promoted to lieutenant colonel. He returned to civilian life at City Sanitarium in 1946. Dr. Moore, his temporary replacement, stepped down to begin private practice, allowing Dr. Kohler to once again dedicate his life to the patients and staff of the sanitarium.

FAREWELL

to the

70th General Hospital

and to

The President of the University,

Lieutenant Chaplain H. B. Crimmins, S.J.

THE FACULTIES OF THE SCHOOLS OF MEDICINE AND DENTISTRY
ST. LOUIS UNIVERSITY

HOTEL STATLER

MONDAY EVENING, DECEMBER 28TH, 1942

6:30 P. M.

Courtesy St. Louis University Archives

"Yesterday is past and over. Tomorrow is unknown, so ... day." —Dr. Kohler, 1961

By 1948 St. Louis City officials had recognized that they could no longer handle the responsibility of City Sanitarium. An offer was made by the State of Missouri to purchase the hospital and land for one dollar. On April 13, 1948, the transfer was made official with the signature of the governor and other state executives. It was agreed that due to his loyal service, as well as his dedication, Dr. Kohler would remain superintendent. Along with new owners came a new name. From that moment on, City Sanitarium would be called St. Louis State Hospital.

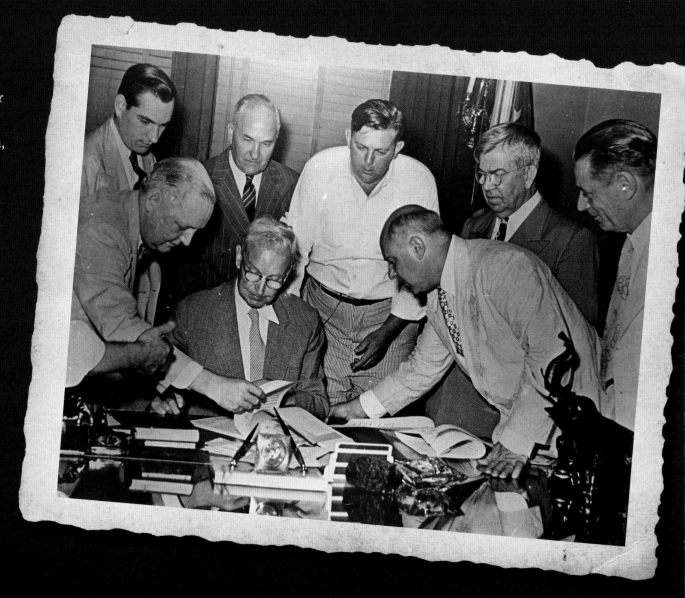

"Encouraging the patient to exercise his self-control, and in firmly, though gently, impressing upon him the necessity of submitting to a healthy discipline, and of accommodating himself to his environment."
—Dr. Howard, 1876

The Bakery

The hospital bakery began as a cost-saving measure during the 1930s. Officials discovered that it was cheaper, and tastier, to make the bread and other sweet treats served at city institutions. City Sanitarium had the room and the patient labor to handle the task. On its busiest days, the bakery supplied goods to both city hospitals and, on special occasions, City Hall. The state's purchase in 1948 ended the burden of baking for the city hospitals but added Malcolm Bliss and St. Louis State School to the roster.

A baker's day began first thing in the morning with getting the prepared bread into the ovens. Once done, the focus turned to breakfast treats such as doughnuts and pastries. It was not uncommon for the bakery team to hand roll, shape, and fry one thousand donuts in a morning. Bread was taken from the oven and sent on its way to be wrapped and shipped. Completed breakfast goods were taken by dietary staff to be served, and the bakers shifted focus once again to the lunch and dinner needs. By mid-afternoon, the bakery staff could relax long enough for their own lunch before beginning preparations for the next morning.

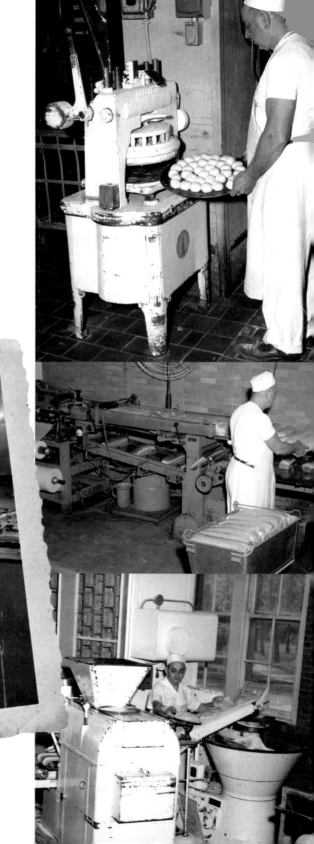

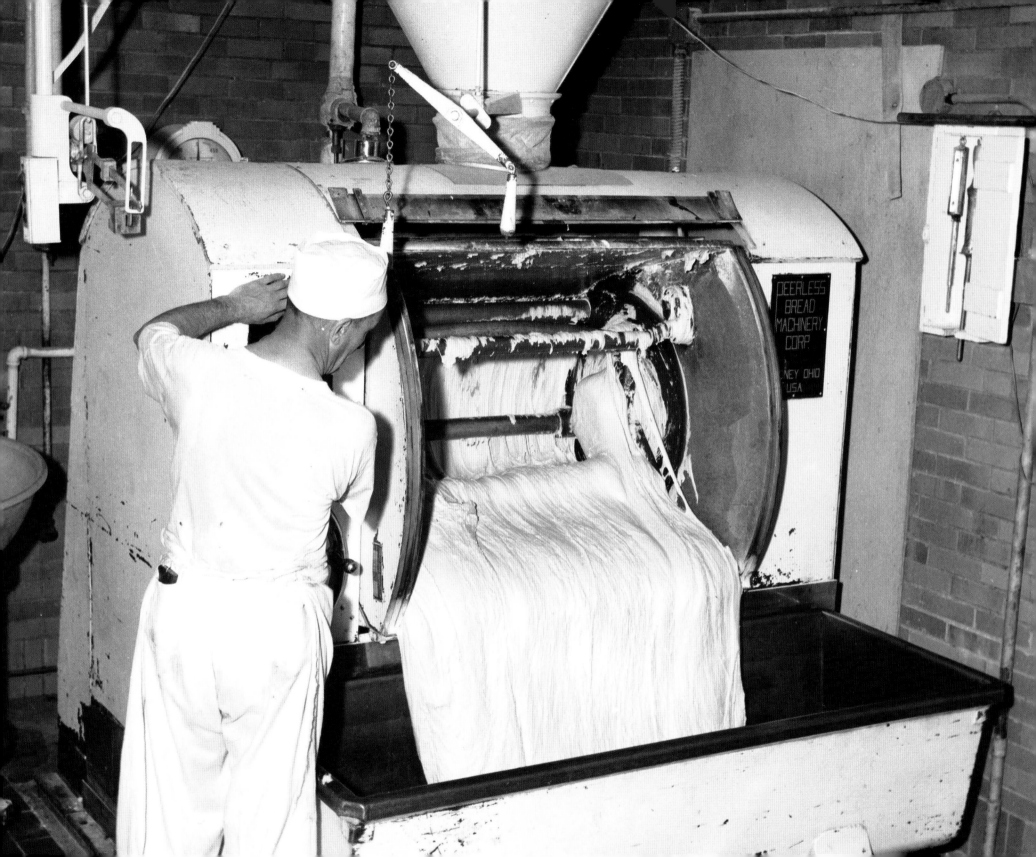

Outpatient Clinic

Since 1900 the constant increases in patient population switched the focus from recovery and return to the community to custodial care. Professionals throughout the state recognized a need for change, but the perpetual funding and staffing shortages impeded progress. Finally, in August 1950 Dr. Kohler, with blessings from Jefferson City officials, opened the St. Louis State Hospital Outpatient Clinic.

The clinic revolutionized mental health care in St. Louis. For the first time, psychiatric services were available to the general public outside an inpatient hospital setting. Clinic services included appointments for psychotherapy, medication services from a psychiatrist, group therapy, and social services referrals for patients with special needs.

As hoped, use of the clinic had an impact on new inpatient admissions by providing alternate means of care for those not in the midst of a crisis. Its popularity also assisted in developing positive relationships with the surrounding community. This in turn broke down certain stereotypes and stigmas associated with mental health and St. Louis State Hospital.

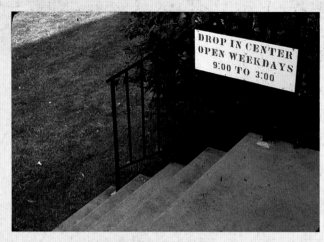

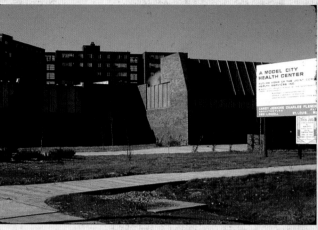

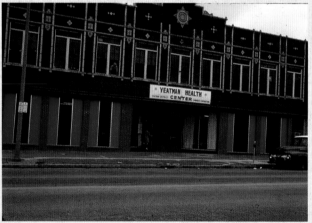

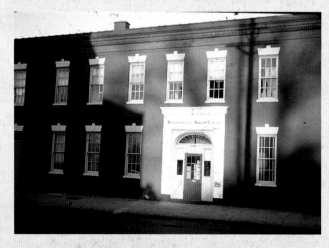

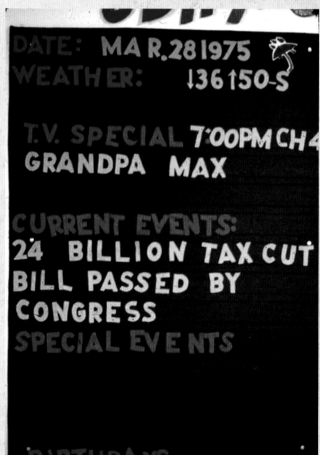

The Compass

The ongoing effort of encouraging patients to be involved in hospital life continued with the creation of *The Compass*. Suggested by Dr. Kohler, the project was initially developed by activity therapy staff and volunteers. They had no problem recruiting interested patients, and regular meetings of what would become known as the Compass Group began.

Together the group decided on the scope, the mission, and, most importantly, the name of the new newspaper. In the spirit of focusing on future recovery, *The Compass* was chosen with the motto "Let the compass point the way." The goal of the paper was to inform patients and staff on the latest hospital developments and to promote communication between wards and programs.

The first issue of *The Compass* newsletter debuted in April 1953. At any given time, paper staff consisted of ten or more patients in various roles. Regular reporters chose topics of interest to the hospital, while the artists and typists focused on the production side of things. Only two staff members were required to assist with printing and

editorial duties. *The Compass* was a hit not only with the hospital, but in the greater community as well. Issues were exchanged with other mental hospitals throughout the country. The paper continued well into the 1960s until, ironically, the skilled individuals responsible for its production were discharged.

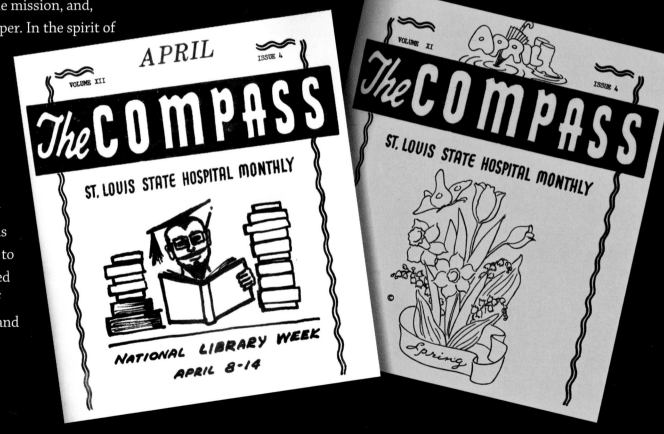

Picnic Time

No matter the financial burdens or struggles, entertainment was always considered an essential part of asylum life. The early days were marked with dances in the fifth-floor ballroom, walks to the park, and various sports on the lawns. In the 1920s, with help and donations from the community, the tradition of the annual picnic was begun.

The picnics of the '20s through the '40s featured games, music, and dancing. The postwar prosperity of the 1950s, plus the ever-growing Auxiliary, raised the picnic to new heights. Rebranded as a carnival, the day began with a parade complete with floats created by each ward. Afterwards patients and staff could enjoy the thrills of the merry-go-round, scrambler, and even pony rides. The Anheuser-Busch Clydesdales made an appearance, along with television and radio personalities. To keep things running smoothly, a committee of employees and volunteers organized the affair, beginning a year in advance. Donations of food, entertainment, and equipment from the community helped make the event affordable without sacrificing any of the fun.

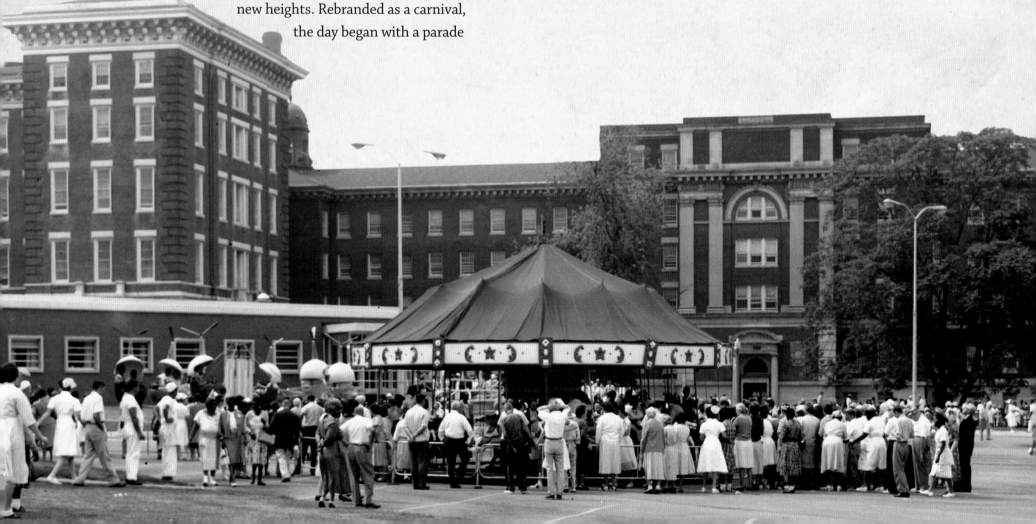

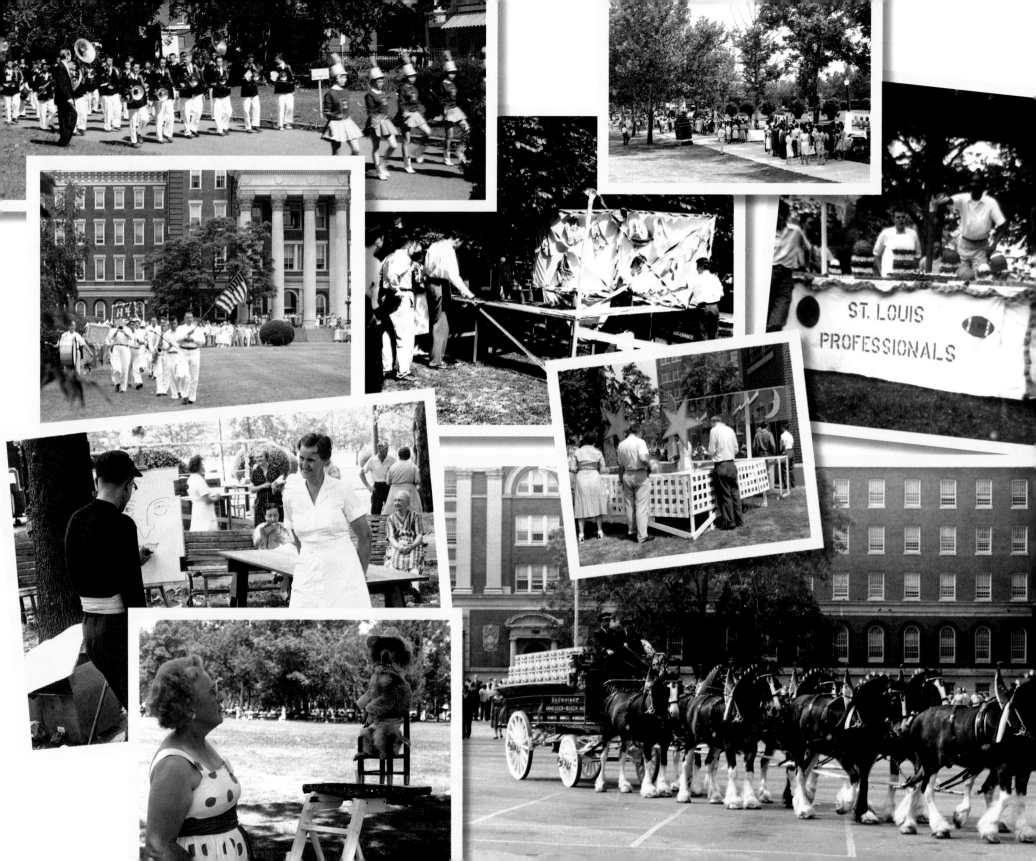

The Auxiliary

From its earliest days, the hospital had relied on the kindness and generosity of the community to supplement everything from entertainment to staff. By the 1950s the postwar optimism and booming economy led to an unprecedented interest in helping out. Dr. Kohler, knowing a good thing when he saw it, organized a Volunteer Services Advisory Committee in early 1953 to act as a liaison between the hospital and interested community members. In February 1954 the Auxiliary of St. Louis State Hospital was born.

The group was formally organized with a board, including the president, vice president, treasurer, and secretary. Other members were welcome to join by paying dues. The Auxiliary and its funds committed itself completely to the welfare of the patients. All fundraisers went directly back into goods and services such as television sets, patient picnics, and new furniture. The group broadcasted its events and meetings through all media available.

In December 1955 their greatest moneymaking achievement was realized with the opening of the hospital canteen. The canteen served every possible treat and sundry to staff, patients, and visitors. It was staffed exclusively by Auxiliary members, and goods were bought at a discount, resulting in almost pure profit. The Auxiliary and its canteen were the first of their kind at Missouri state hospitals, and the Auxiliary's example went on to influence how communities and volunteers were utilized throughout the mental health system.

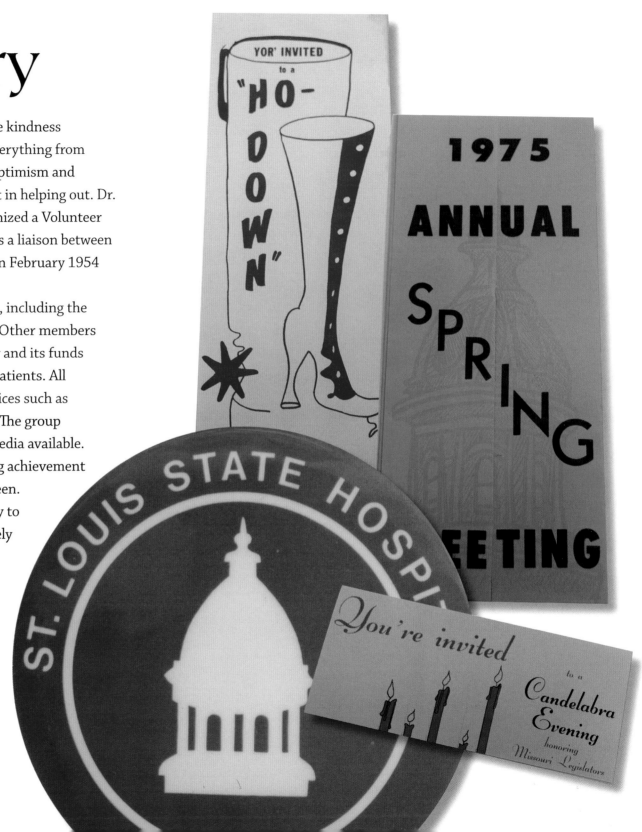

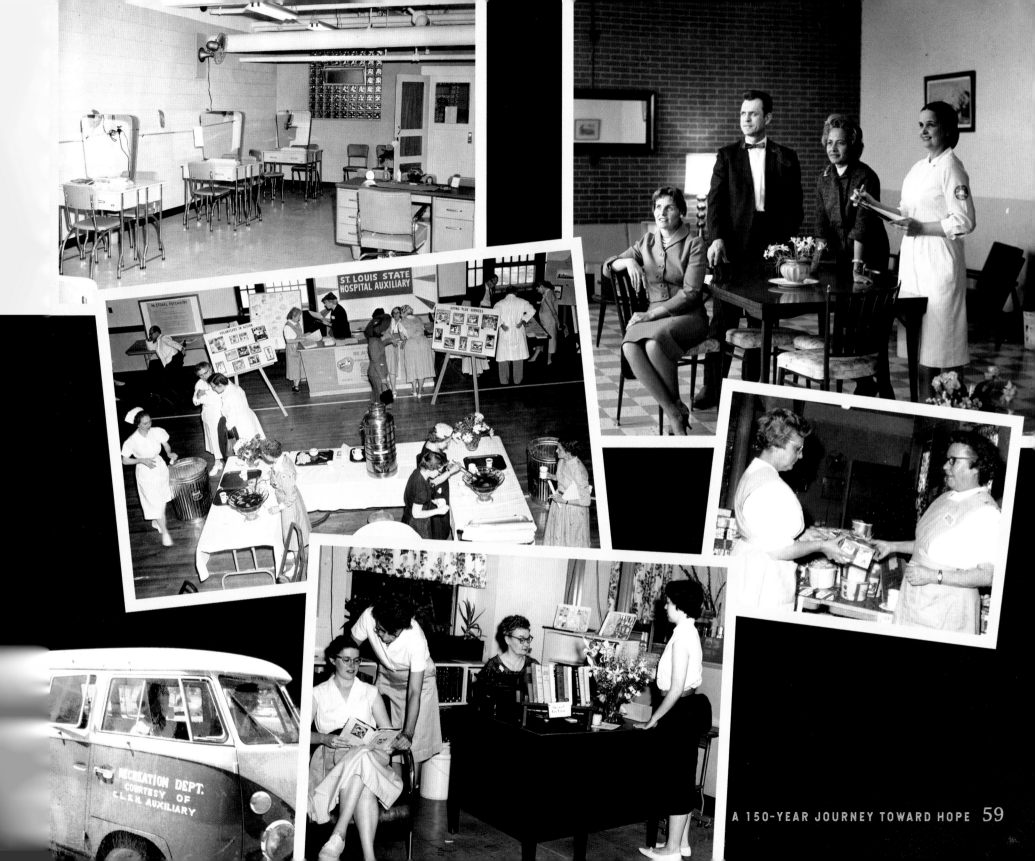

Christmas Caroling

The November through February nursing classes found themselves at the San for both Thanksgiving and Christmas. For many of them, this meant an extra dose of homesickness. Miss Gulmi and Miss Bigler decided to combat the issue by keeping the students busy providing a little something extra for the patients.

On Christmas morning students were expected to arrive in the dorm recreation room by 4 a.m. dressed in full uniform. Miss Gulmi handed everyone a pair of red taper candles. Lining up two by two, the students headed out of their residence and into the sleeping hospital. Candles were lit as they entered the building. Guided only by their flames, the students began walking through the corridors singing "Silent Night."

Two hours later, the group had wound its way through all fifty-two halls, bringing the official start to Christmas for the patients and staff. After attending Christmas Mass in the auditorium, the group reconvened in the employees' dining room for a hearty breakfast. Instructors surprised the students with small gifts and trinkets. When everyone had eaten their fill, they headed off to their ward assignments to spend an unforgettable Christmas away from home.

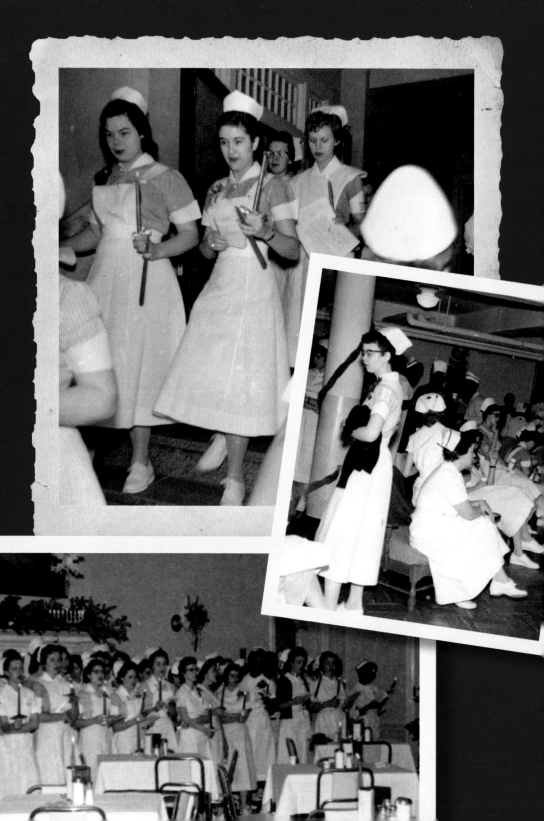

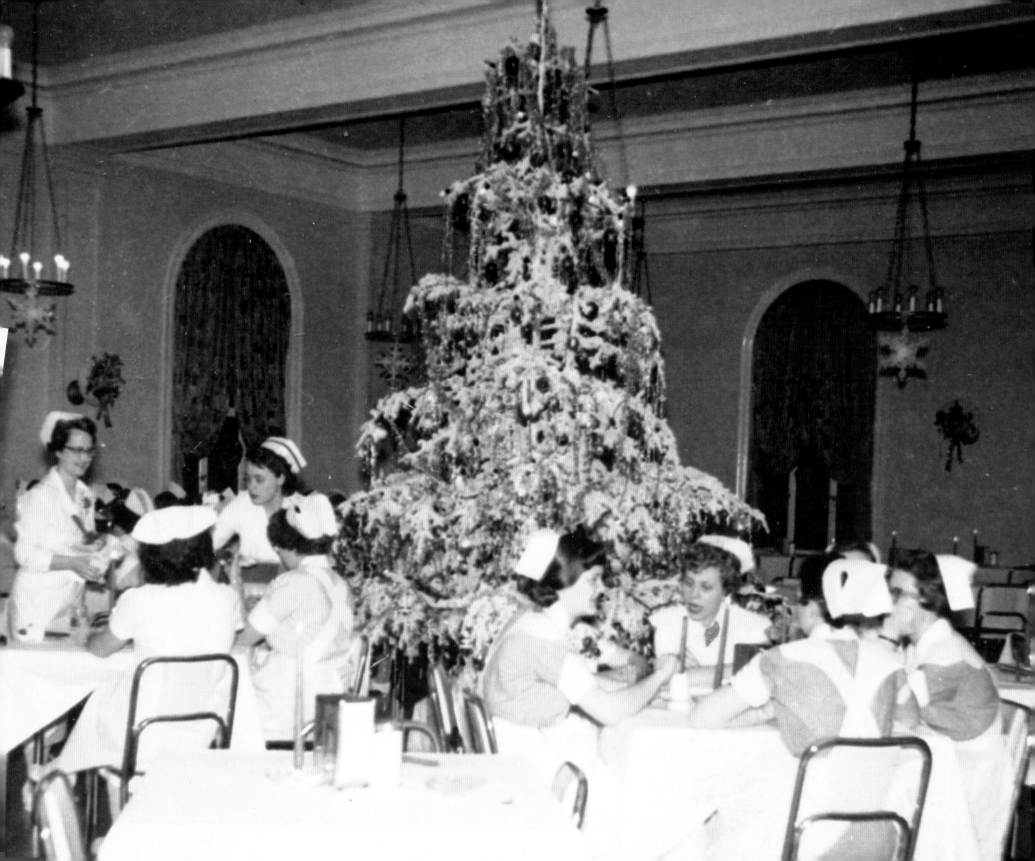

Mr. Jingle and the Belles

In November 1953 the nursing education department made history as Mr. Blount, the first male student nurse, started classes. Blount arrived with the affiliate class from General Hospital in Kansas City. He took part in the publicity committee and was known as the errand boy. As a tribute to his status, the scrapbook committee named their volume "Mr. Jingle and the Belles."

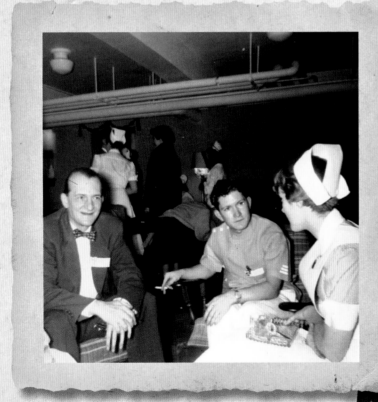

Mr. Blount and Dr. Busch

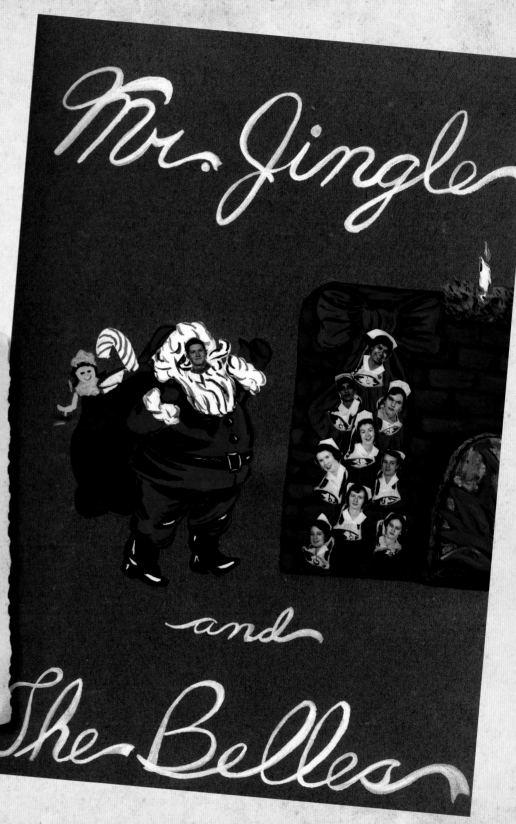

Growing Affiliations

By 1950 Dr. Kohler had been serving as superintendent for almost a decade. During this time he had become increasingly aware of the constant staffing struggles and related patient care issues. Taking inspiration from the success of the student nurse program, he decided to investigate psychiatric affiliations with other disciplines. These relationships would serve a dual purpose. On one hand, graduate students would be able to fulfill practicum requirements, while on the other, the hospital would benefit from the supplemental staffing.

In July 1950 the first psychiatric social work students were sent from the George Warren Brown School at Washington University. Each of the ten students was placed on a ward to provide social services to patients and gain experience working with doctors, nurses, and attendants. This "thrown in

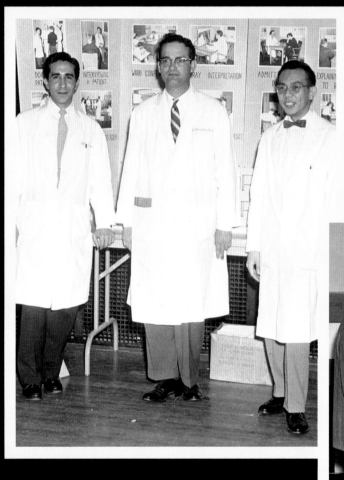

the deep end" approach was surprisingly effective and popular. The school of social work at St. Louis University heard of the experiment and asked to be included but, due to space issues, had to be put off for an additional year.

The most exciting development occurred in March 1951 when the American Medical Association approved St. Louis State Hospital as a residency site for psychiatry. As part of the AMA's terms, residents would be required to spend three years at the hospital providing direct care to patients. Once again, the use of students would provide multiple benefits.

Open House

As public awareness of mental illness grew, so did the need to invite the community to see the hospital they helped fund. Open House Day was officially established in 1950 to provide this opportunity. Planning began a year in advance, with committees of committees to handle every aspect. Each year had a different theme, ranging from "Open House" to "Hospital Careers: An Opportunity to Serve." Displays from every department and discipline were set up in the auditorium, with the Auxiliary serving refreshments. Student nurses and interested staff gave tours of the hospital, while doctors stood by to answer questions. Lasting all day, Open House Day would have up to one thousand visitors, thanks to interest and advertising in local media.

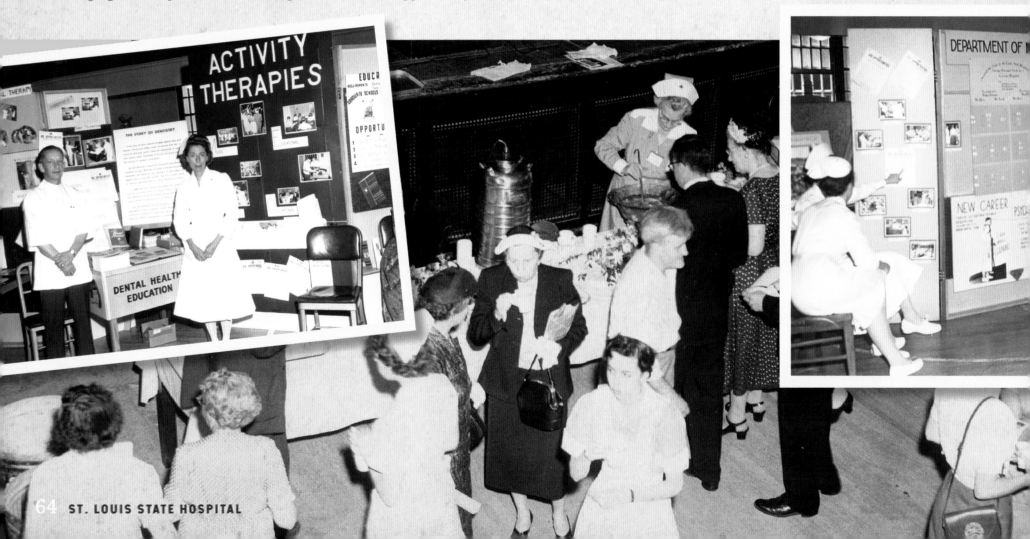

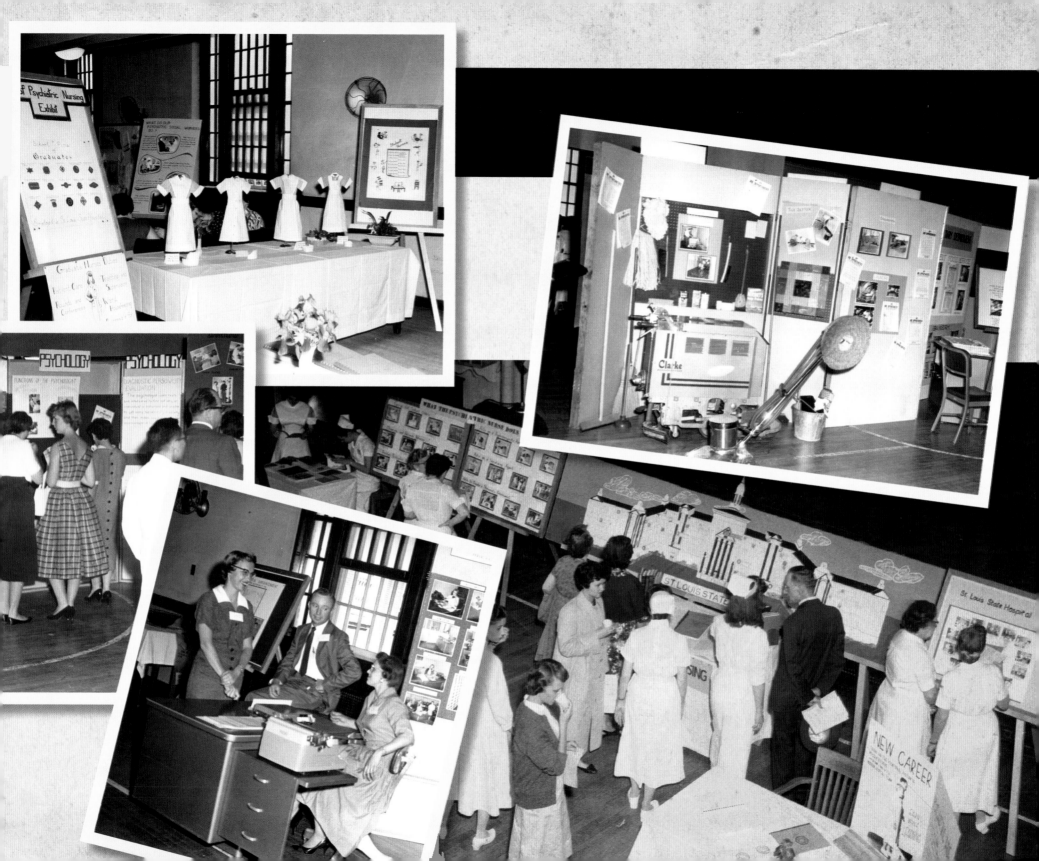

Portrait of an Aide

In his 1896 report to the mayor, Dr. Runge called for the creation of an attendant training program. He believed that in order to properly care for patients, attendants needed to learn the basic skills of anatomy and psychology. He also felt that by investing the time and effort of teaching in the attendants, they would feel valued and be more likely to remain with the hospital.

In 1929 assistant superintendent Dr. Kohler instituted a training program for attendants. This initial program was designed to last three months and consisted of a series of lectures. It proved popular with the staff, but the struggles of the 1930s and the outbreak of World War II interrupted its progress.

Finally, in February 1950 Dr. Kohler was able to return to his dream, and the first class of psychiatric aides began that month. Dr. Kohler, registered nurse Viola Laurent, and student nurse instructor Dillie Gulmi worked together to create a comprehensive, yearlong curriculum.

While geared toward hospital attendants, all employees were invited to apply to the school. Included in the application process was a psychological exam, a basic reading and writing test, and a physical. Those chosen needed to be prepared to dedicate a year to their studies and to live on campus with the student nurses.

The first class consisted of twenty attendants. Taking a cue from the student nurses, that first group documented their year and their progress in a scrapbook. Their training consisted of lectures as well as clinical opportunities. Occasionally, psychiatric aide students would learn side by side with nursing students.

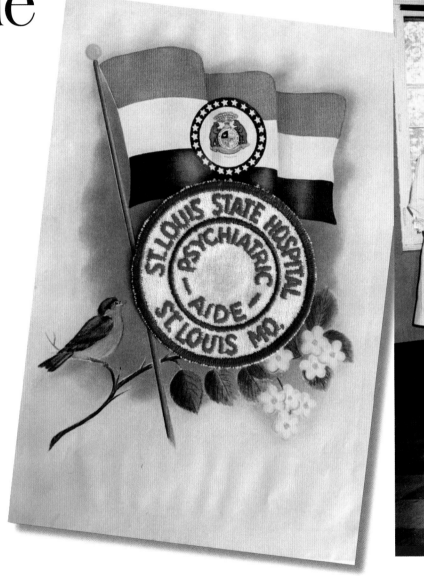

"No greater pleasure can be experienced than to see a human soul emerge from the pit of utter despair."
—*Dr. Runge, 1901*

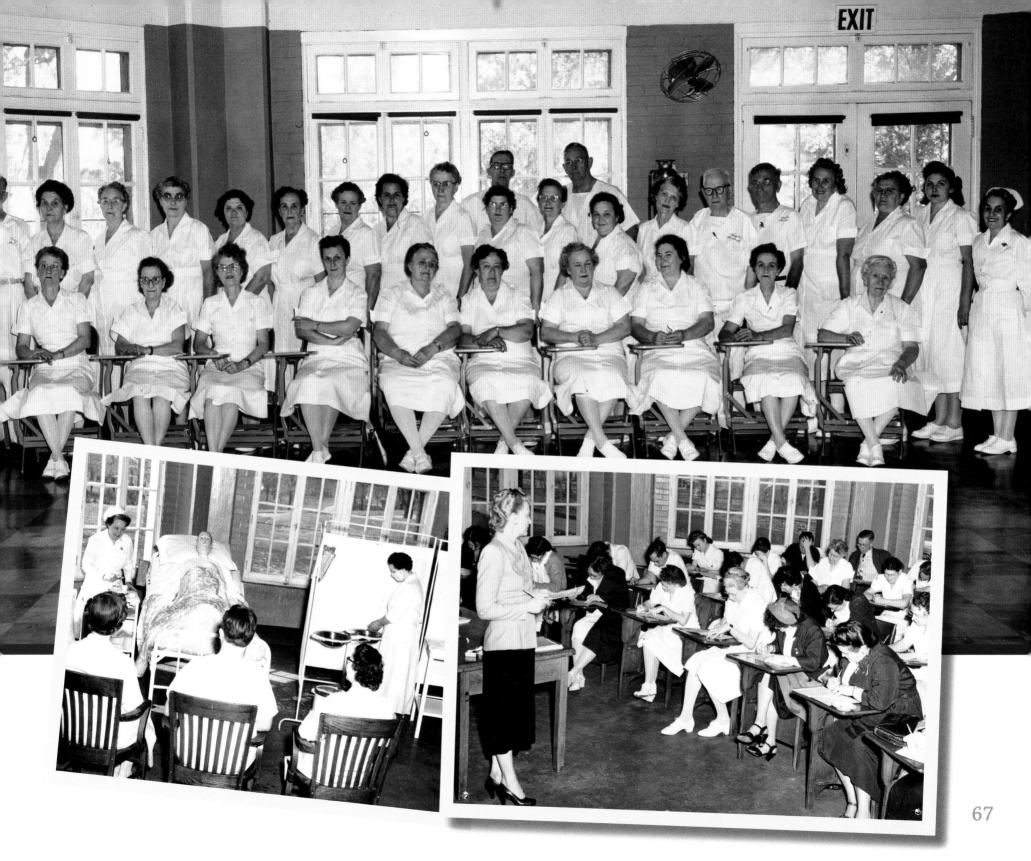

Psychiatric Aide Graduation

On March 15, 1951, more than one hundred people gathered in the St. Louis State Hospital auditorium for the graduation of the first psychiatric aide class. Family, friends, and patients watched as the new aides received a diploma from Dr. Kohler and a pin from director of education Miss Bigler. Completion of the course gave graduates a new title, a job classification (created especially for the program), and uniforms. Male psychiatric aides wore starched white pants, a shirt, and polished white shoes, with a black belt and bowtie. Female aides' uniforms consisted of white tights, polished white shoes, and a starched white dress. Both men and women wore a psychiatric aide green, red, and white "St. Louis State Hospital, Psychiatric Aide" patch on their left shoulder.

The program was the first of its kind in Missouri. From all accounts it was an instant success. Enrollment for the second class was filled before the first had finished and it was not uncommon for there to be a waiting list for applicants. The training classes continued well into the 1970s and, as Dr. Runge predicted, produced long-term and valuable employees.

Portrait of an Aide, Sterling Conway, 1951

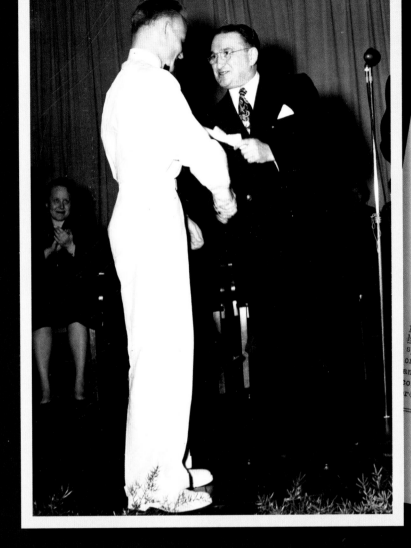

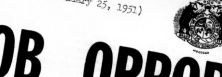

Official Public Notice
Please Post

JOB OPPORTUNITIES

THE PERSONNEL DIVISION OF MISSOURI

Announces Examination for

PSYCHIATRIC AIDE I

PSYCHIATRIC AIDE II

This examination is <u>promotional</u> and open only to employees of the St. Louis State Hospital who meet the necessary requirements.

Psychiatric Aide I — Salary $178-227

<u>DUTIES</u>: This is sub-professional psychiatric and general nursing work in the care and treatment of mentally and physically ill patients in a mental hospital. <u>MINIMUM EXPERIENCE AND TRAINING QUALIFICATIONS</u>: Completion of the eighth school grade; and graduation from the one-year basic training program for Psychiatric Aides as conducted at the St. Louis State Hospital, or graduation from a comparable training program for Psychiatric Aides.

Psychiatric Aide II — Salary $206-262

<u>DUTIES</u>: This is responsible sub-professional psychiatric and general nursing work involving the supervision of a large number of subordinate attendants and Psychiatric Aides engaged in the care and treatment of mentally and physically ill patients in a mental hospital. <u>MINIMUM EXPERIENCE AND TRAINING QUALIFICATIONS</u>: Three years of progressively responsible experience in the hospital care of mental patients, including at least one year in a charge capacity on a ward; and completion of the tenth school grade and graduation from the one-year basic training program for Psychiatric Aides as conducted at the St. Louis State Hospital, or graduation from a comparable training program for Psychiatric Aides.

APPLICATIONS

Must be on the Official Form and Postmarked by Midnight of

February 10, 1951

"No community may boast of having even approached the standard of perfection unless it is able to show, during the course of its normal development, an honest and unremitting endeavor of solving those problems in accordance with the dictates of modern sociologic science and of true philanthropy, and, whenever and wherever feasible, of aiming at the prevention of numerical growth of the dependent and afflicted classes, inclusive of the insane." —Dr. Runge, 1901

Summer of Sports

The summer of 1961 was a busy one for St. Louis State Hospital sports fans. In June San Francisco Giants center fielder Willie Mays paid a visit to patients and staff. Fans gathered on the softball field behind the main building for a motivational talk from the star player, followed by a hitting exhibition. A recreational therapist filled in as pitcher, while the balls were fielded by members of the patients' softball team.

A few weeks later, St. Louis Cardinals' manager Johnny Keane and star player Joe Cunningham stopped by to give a baseball clinic. Again, a large crowd of fans gathered around the diamond to hear them speak. Afterwards Keane and Cunningham demonstrated plays for the softball team and gave them tips.

The summer of sports wrapped up with a visit from the St. Louis Hawks basketball team. It was standing room only in the auditorium as the Hawks demonstrated basic shots, ball feeding, and handling. Afterwards the Hawks took on the St. Louis State Hospital Squad in a brief game. Using the new tricks and tips, the patients' team held their own with the pros and made the hospital proud.

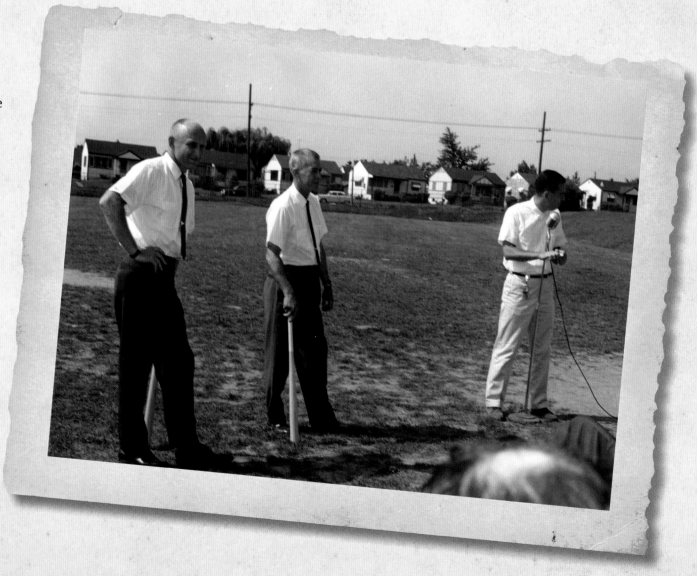

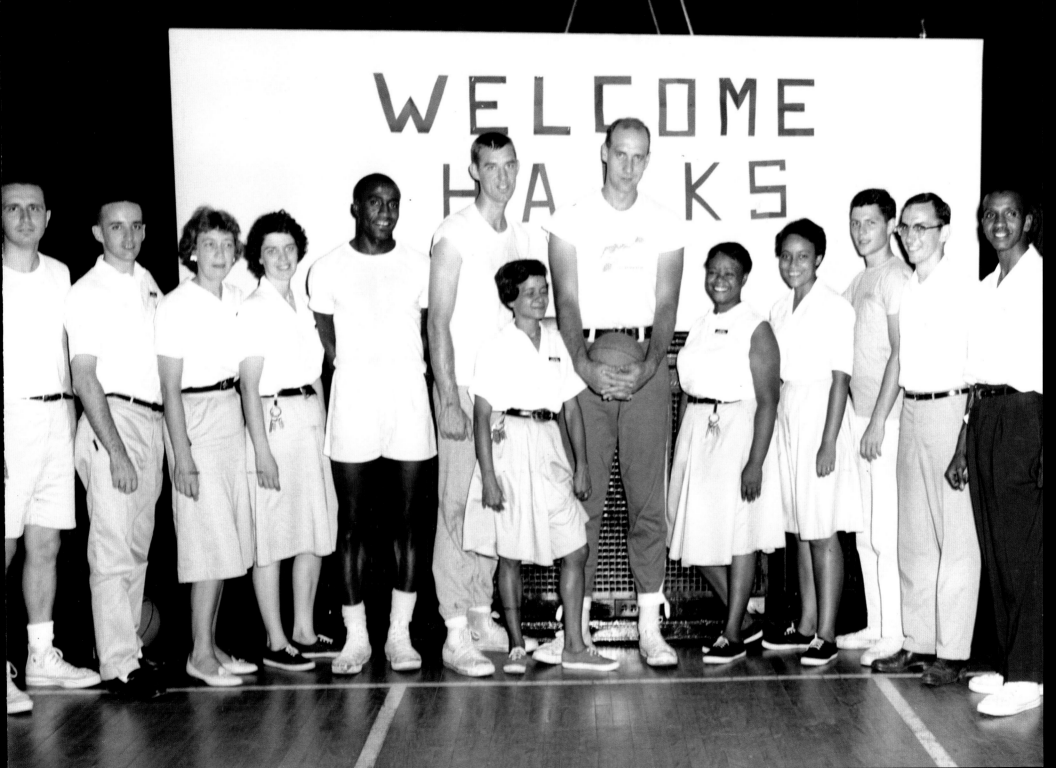

St. Louis State Hospital. Originally affiliated with the Washington University School of Medicine, the institute underwent a series of changes until it ultimately became part of the University of Missouri system. Institute staff provided experience and training to medical students interested in psychiatry according to the best practices at the time. In the spirit of scholarship, the institute hired a professional librarian to develop a world-class collection of texts relevant to psychiatry and mental health.

The new facility was housed in a state-of-the-art building constructed and designed in mid-century modern style. While the building was originally intended to be four stories, budget issues. The contractors in charge of the elevators did not receive the message in time, however, and elevator shafts were left to poke out of the roof. This oversight resulted in completion of the four floors, if for no other reason than to fix the eyesore. By the end of the 1960s, it was decided to add on two more floors to house a new computer lab and research area. Unfortunately, the weight of the 1960s computer equipment placed on the top floor of the building led to significant structural damage, ensuring the demolition of the building in later years.

In tribute to his forward thinking, long career, and love of research, the new building was christened after Dr. Louis Kohler on October 22, 1962.

EXECUTIVE OFFICE
STATE OF MISSOURI
JEFFERSON CITY

JOHN M. DALTON
GOVERNOR

September 7, 1962

Mr. Russell W. Sexton, Chairman
Mental Health Commission
722 Jefferson Street
Jefferson City, Missouri

Dear Russ:

I appreciated receiving your letter of August 31st regarding the idea of naming the new building at the St. Louis State Hospital in honor of Dr. Louis H. Kohler.

Of course, I think this is an excellent suggestion and I think the idea of making it a surprise announcement on the day of dedication is fine.

With best personal regards, I am

Sincerely yours,

Governor

August 31, 1962

Honorable John M. Dalton
Governor, State of Missouri
Capitol Building
Jefferson City, Missouri

Dear Governor Dalton:

At the meeting of the State Mental Health Commission on August 23, 1962, it was approved, subject to your wishes, that the new building at the St. Louis State Hospital be named in honor of Louis H. Kohler, M.D. who has given his life's work to developing this hospital.

We wondered if you might wish to keep this as a surprise and announce it on the day of the dedication.

Sincerely yours,

Russell W. Sexton
Chairman
Mental Health Commission

Governor John M. Dalton

Requests Your Presence at the Dedication

of

The Newly Established Training and
Research Facility

The Missouri Institute of Psychiatry

of

The St. Louis State Hospital
5400 Arsenal Street
Saint Louis 39, Missouri

2:00 P. M. O'clock
Monday, October 22, 1962

Speaker: Jack R. Ewalt, Jr., M. D.
Professor of Psychiatry
Harvard University

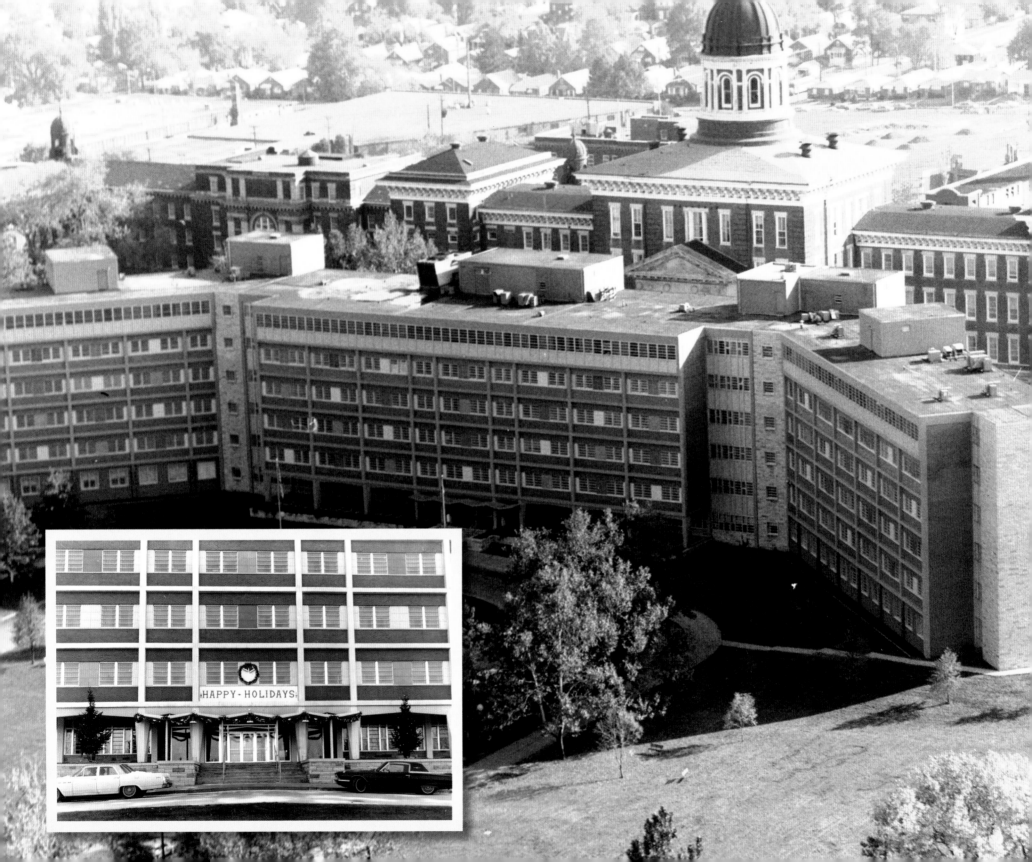

HAPPY·HOLIDAYS

A Year of Fires

Despite making significant strides in decreasing the patient population, in 1965 the hospital was still home to 2,600 patients. It was not unusual to find sixty residents in a ward designed for a maximum of thirty. Staffing issues, especially at night, continued to make it difficult to maintain an adequate level of supervision. These issues would lead to tragedy on the night of January 15.

At approximately 9:20 p.m., an attendant on Ward C-3 smelled smoke during her evening rounds. She immediately alerted the switchboard as the automatic smoke alarm began to sound. Evacuation of the entire west wing was underway when the first firetruck arrived. Student nurses, having just learned fire drill procedures four hours earlier, ran across campus to assist. While the grounds filled with 1,200 female patients, fire consumed the third floor and threatened the second and fourth.

The fifth fire alarm was sounded at 9:50 p.m., and the fire was declared under control by 10:15 p.m. By this time, more than 175 firemen, twenty pumpers, six hook and ladders, and five hose wagons were on the scene. Fighting the blaze was nearly impossible because of the secure metal bars on each window. Firemen were forced to break through glass and drag hoses up stairwells to get to the fire.

When it was safe to enter, firemen discovered two patients on either side of the ward where they had attempted to hide from the fire. Physicians tried to provide medical care, but the women were declared dead at the scene. Considering the number of patients, lack of escape routes, and difficulty getting to the blaze, it was incredibly fortunate that more lives were not lost.

The fire marshal later determined that the fire had begun in a clothing room. The linens and toilet paper caught quickly. By the time the attendant had smelled smoke, the fire was well under way. It was thought, but never proven, that a forgotten cigarette was the cause.

1965

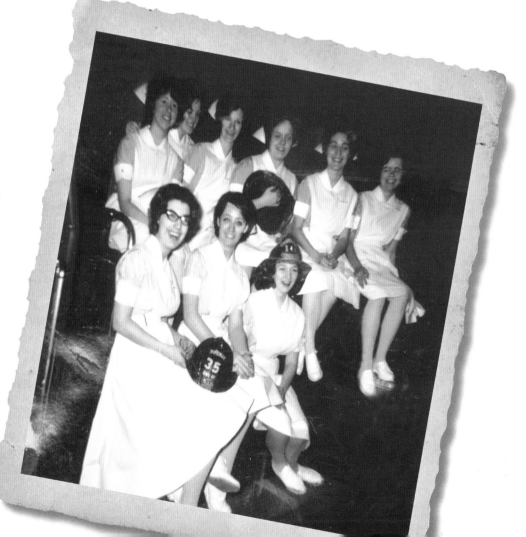

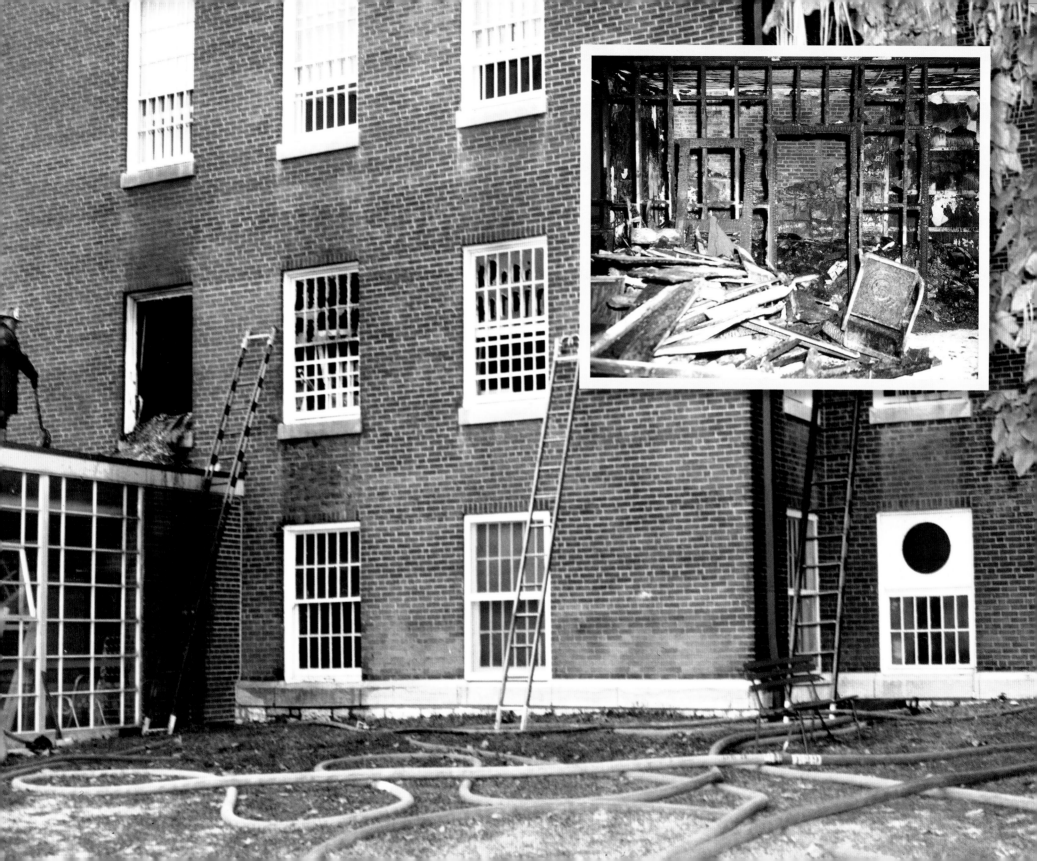

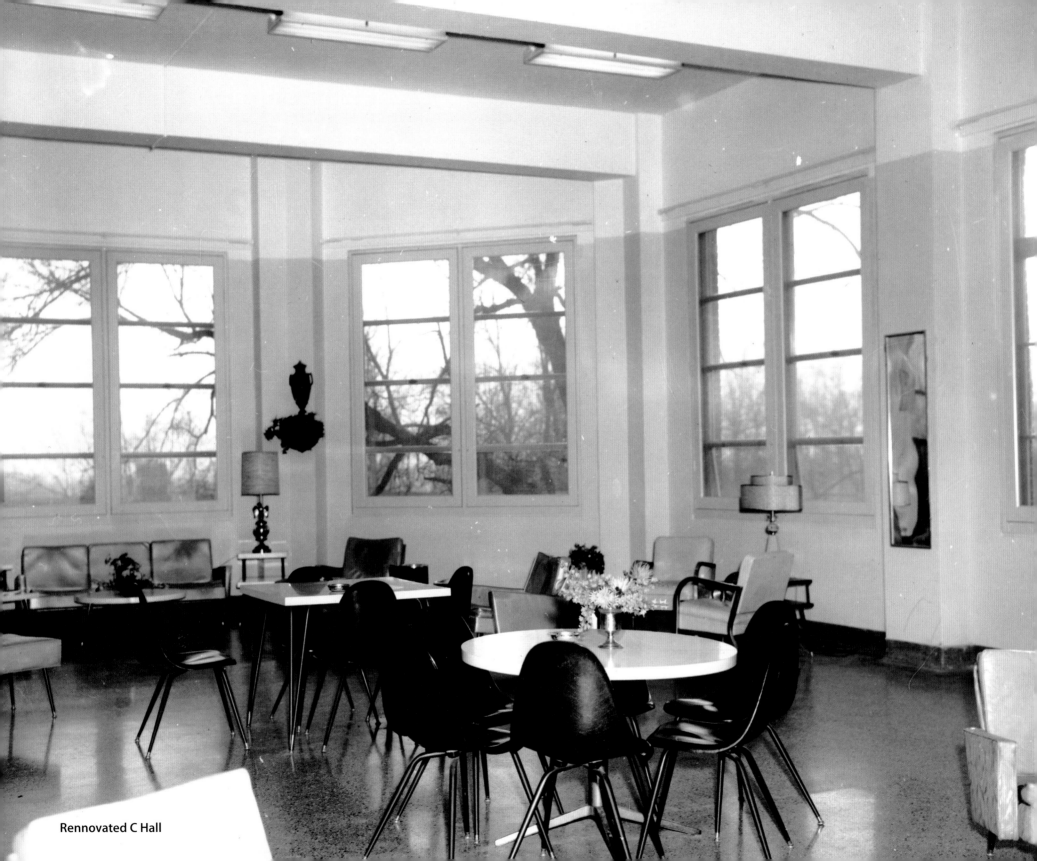

Rennovated C Hall

Arsonist on C-0

The hospital was still recovering from the January tragedy when a series of mysterious fires broke out in early November. Within a twenty-four-hour period, Ward C-0 experienced three separate—and thankfully small—blazes. Fast-acting staff were able to contain each one before significant damage could be done. Nevertheless, patients from C-0, as well as neighboring D-0, were evacuated. A full investigation by the St. Louis City arson squad determined that a patient was to blame.

In the aftermath, state officials funded several projects to protect the building from future incidents. Wooden shelving was replaced with fireproof steel lockers in all of the ward clothing rooms and linen closets. Additional smoke detectors and fire extinguishers were purchased. Finally, the entire building was fitted with an up-to-date sprinkler system.

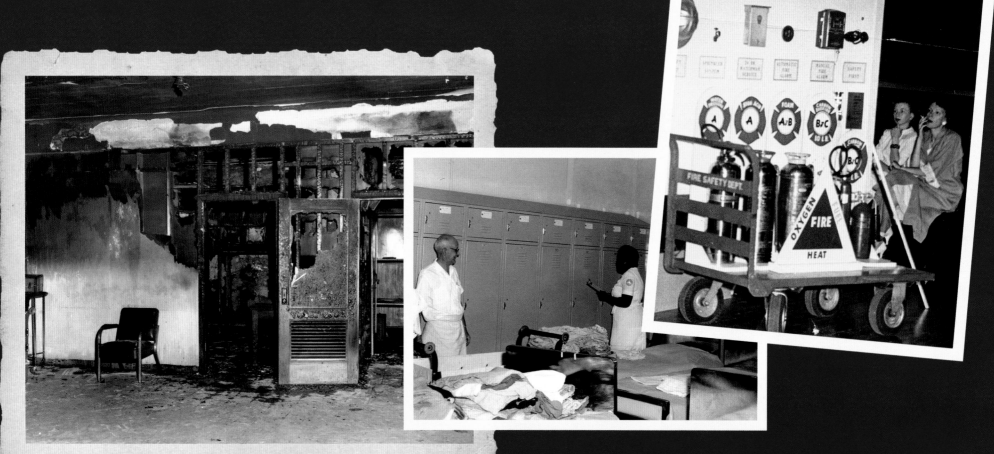

The Outlook

In 1964 a group of volunteers decided to confront the stigma surrounding mental illness and the state hospital head on. Working with the hospital community relations staff, the seven women developed *The Outlook*. The quarterly magazine highlighted the "spirit of dedication" contained within the gates on Arsenal by featuring events, people, and treatments. Unlike other internal publications, *The Outlook* was designed to be read by the community. Copies of each issue were printed by the thousands and distributed by mail and foot to interested parties.

To make things easier on the original seven, staff members with news to share could write up their own articles and be listed as "contributing editors." Each issue came in at around twenty pages and contained numerous photos to accompany the stories. *The Outlook* was published faithfully for almost a decade before the task became too time consuming for the elderly volunteers. Later issues appeared intermittently through the 1970s and '80s, but it was never the same.

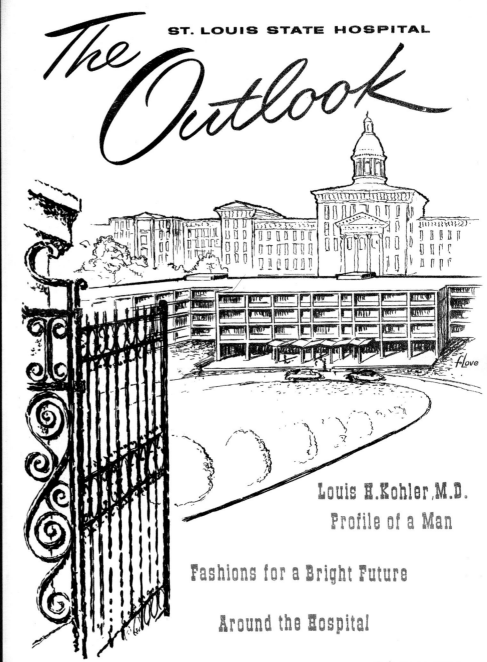

ST. LOUIS STATE HOSPITAL

The Outlook

Louis H. Kohler, M.D.
Profile of a Man

Fashions for a Bright Future

Around the Hospital

February 1964

Employees' Bulletin

Following the success of *The Outlook*, Dr. Knowles decided that the more than one thousand hospital employees needed an internal counterpart. On October 27, 1965, Flo Kinyon, head of community relations, debuted the *Employees' Bulletin*. Known almost immediately as simply the *Bulletin*, the weekly publication was designed strictly for internal information. Generally no more than four pages long, the *Bulletin* contained items such as reminders from administration, new employees, updated phone numbers, and other tidbits. Unlike *The Outlook*, it rarely featured photographs and was always produced by a staff member.

The *Bulletin* would appear in several versions over the years, including a brief period as a daily publication, but it always remained in one form or another. In the pre-email era, it provided up-to-date information on hospital activities and issues. In 1997 the *Bulletin* underwent yet another change to correspond with the opening of the new hospital buildings. Rebranded *The Pulse*, it continued to keep staff and patients in the know.

Employees **SLSH** Bulletin

R.R.Knowles, M.D., Sup't.   October 27, 1965   F.L. Kinyon, Editor

Each month St. Louis State Hospital receives many newsletters from other hospitals and organizations. We feel the need now of a Bulletin of our own to acquaint our 1,300 employees with news of our hospital. We all do a better job when we are well-informed. It is true that we already have a very effective grapevine method of spreading information (and misinformation), but this method has disadvantages, not the least that it is not authoritative. We hope this news report will be more reliable. It should be pointed out that it will serve a different function to Outlook; our circulation is restricted and our goal is to acquaint our personnel with the hospital's policies, problems and programs.

All employees are invited to contribute to these columns. Questions may be raised or answers offered to the questions others raise. We will endeavor to answer honestly those appropriate to this Bulletin.

SOCIAL WORK STUDENTS ASSIGNED

The following social service students from Washington University are assigned to Section IV until next May: Donald Roy Bice, Miss Patricia Browder, Miss Elizabeth Davis, Mrs. Patricia McTaggart, Mrs. Dorothy McMurtry, Robert Dean Nowlin, Miss LaNell Schade.

The students from St. Louis University are working on Section Z. They are: Miss Patricia Quinlan, Charles Lee, Sister Mary Eugenia Ponzini, Mrs. Elsie Witt, Rev. Joseph Buckley, Kenneth Leibrich.

- - - - -

The former Miss Barbara Bronn, social worker in the Outpatient Clinic is now Mrs. R. Alan Murray.

Miss Earline Ingram, P.S.W., is now the Family Care Worker. Her station is 213.

UNITED FUND CAMPAIGN

Two heartwarming things happened during the United Fund Campaign -- One of our patients contributed one cent, which may have been the largest gift of all. And an employee wrote us: "I am on vacation going thru Texas on way to New Mexico tomorrow. But I did want to contribute to United Fund and feared your records might be closed when I get back. Hope this is OK." Enclosed was this wonderful person's contribution.

Dr. Cecil G. Baker, Assistant Superintendent, has just been appointed Associate Professor in the Department of Psychiatry at St. Louis University Medical School.

Outfits, Ltd.

One of the first Auxiliary projects was the matter of patient clothing. Up until this point, patients with no relatives and no money were provided with clothing made in the hospital sewing room. While the clothes were nice enough, they did not lend themselves to special occasions. As the hospital focus began shifting away from custodial care to the community, Auxiliary members recognized a need for access to finer things.

Outfits, Ltd., was designed as a one-stop shopping destination. With the help of Auxiliary stylists, male and female patients could assemble an entire outfit. The newly dapper residents were now prepared for job interviews, community trips, and visits with relatives.

Originally housed in the basement, by the 1960s Outfits, Ltd., had moved to a place of honor in the fifth-floor round room. Mrs. Ruth Meyer, chairman of the project, spent several months scouring the hospital for antique furniture. With the help of patient workers, cabinets and bookcases were painted in stylish colors and converted into "practical and charming shelf space." A "gaily" painted trunk was filled with purses and a hat bar allowed patients to "select a becoming chapeau." Gentlemen visitors could browse the tie rack and choose cuff links or belts.

Displaying the chicest fashions of the day was Gertie the Mannequin. Standing in the center of the room, Gertie greeted and inspired shoppers daily.

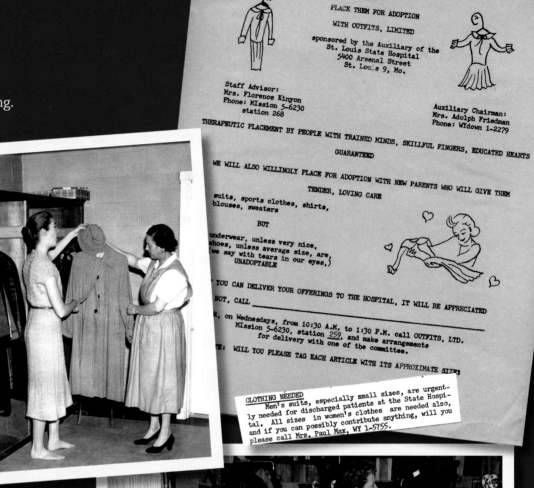

DOES A DRESS OF YOURS FEEL REJECTED IN THE CLOSET ???

IS YOUR GOOD, CLEAN OLD COAT SUFFERING FROM INFERIORITY FEELINGS ???

PLACE THEM FOR ADOPTION

WITH OUTFITS, LIMITED

sponsored by the Auxiliary of the
St. Louis State Hospital
5400 Arsenal Street
St. Louis 9, Mo.

Staff Advisor:
Mrs. Florence Kinyon
Phone: MIssion 5-6230
station 268

Auxiliary Chairman:
Mrs. Adolph Friedman
Phone: WYdown 1-2279

THERAPEUTIC PLACEMENT BY PEOPLE WITH TRAINED MINDS, SKILLFUL FINGERS, EDUCATED HEARTS
GUARANTEED

WE WILL ALSO WILLINGLY PLACE FOR ADOPTION WITH NEW PARENTS WHO WILL GIVE THEM
TENDER, LOVING CARE

suits, sports clothes, shirts,
blouses, sweaters

BUT

underwear, unless very nice,
shoes, unless average size, are,
(we say with tears in our eyes,)
UNADOPTABLE

IF YOU CAN DELIVER YOUR OFFERINGS TO THE HOSPITAL, IT WILL BE APPRECIATED

IF NOT, CALL _____

OR, on Wednesdays, from 10:30 A.M. to 1:30 P.M. call OUTFITS, LTD.
MIssion 5-6230, station 259, and make arrangements
for delivery with one of the committee.

NOTE: WILL YOU PLEASE TAG EACH ARTICLE WITH ITS APPROXIMATE SIZE?

CLOTHING NEEDED
Men's suits, especially small sizes, are urgent-
ly needed for discharged patients at the State Hospital. All sizes in women's clothes are needed also,
and if you can possibly contribute anything, will you
please call Mrs. Paul Max, WY 1-5755.

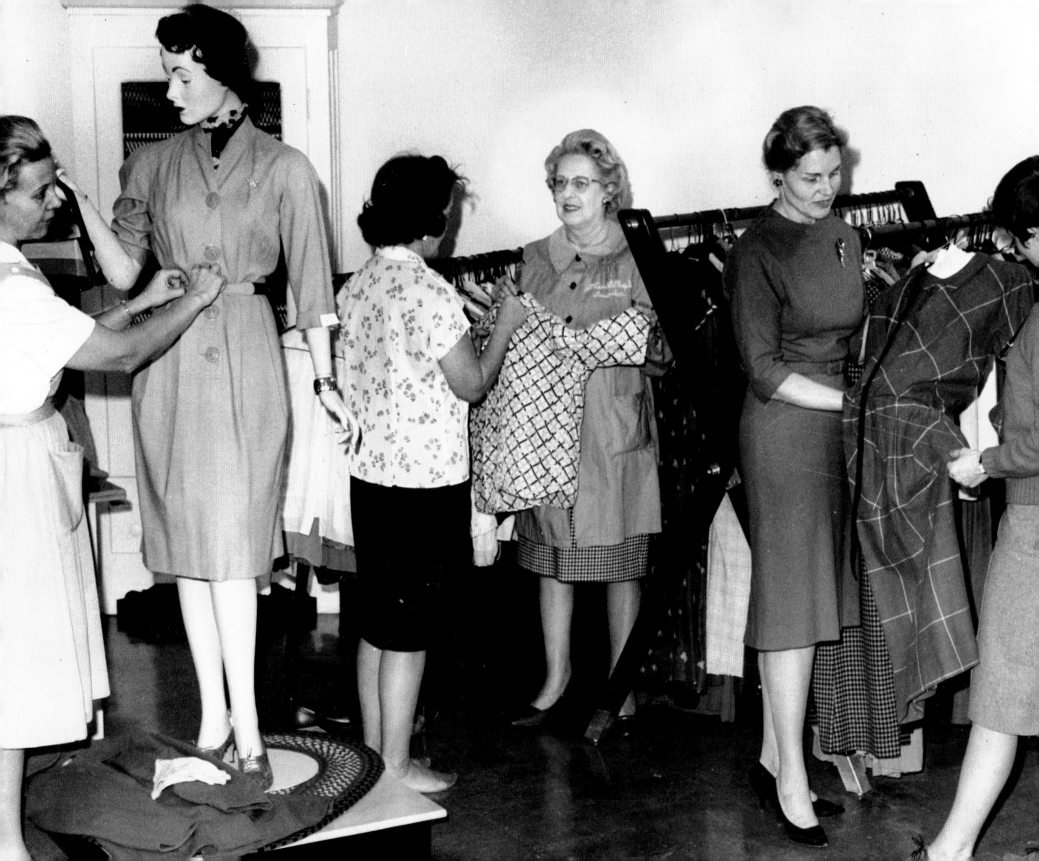

In and Out Shop

While Outfits, Ltd., met the need for formalwear, everyday clothes were available in the In and Out Shop. Prior to the shift in treatment toward rehabilitation in the 1950s, indigent patients received clothes from the sewing room as needed. After changing focus to encourage recovery and discharge, hospital administration and the occupational therapy department saw an opportunity to provide patients with real-world experience. Custom cabinetry from the carpenter shop plus new curtains and plenty of elbow grease transformed a large basement space into a miniature department store. Unlike the collection of donated finer items at Outfits, Ltd., the In and Out Shop featured the items made by the sewing room in an attractive environment. Though different in purpose, both stores allowed patients to choose their own clothes and get a taste of the shopping experience.

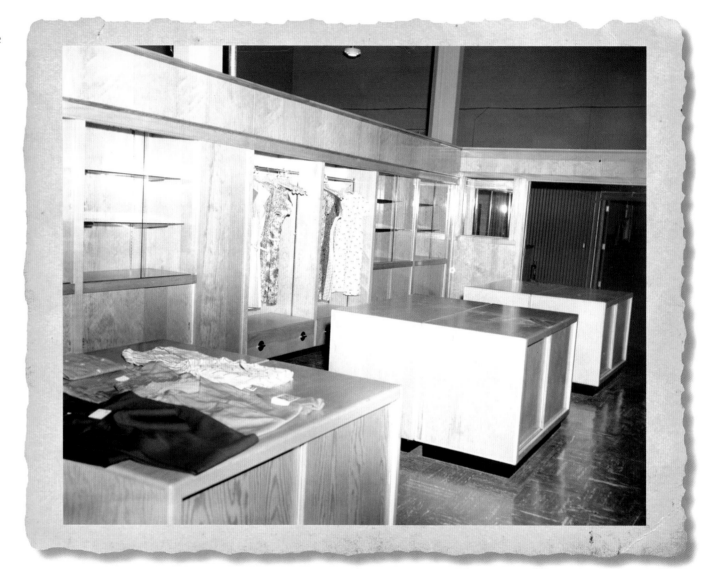

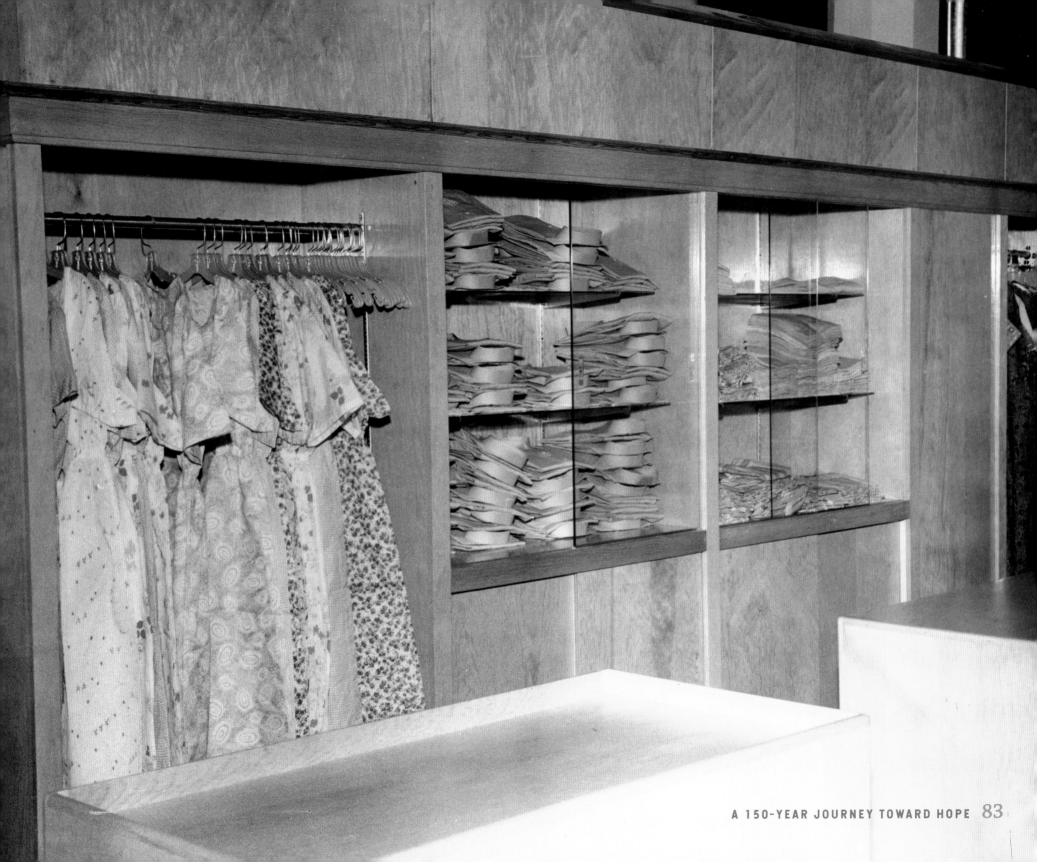

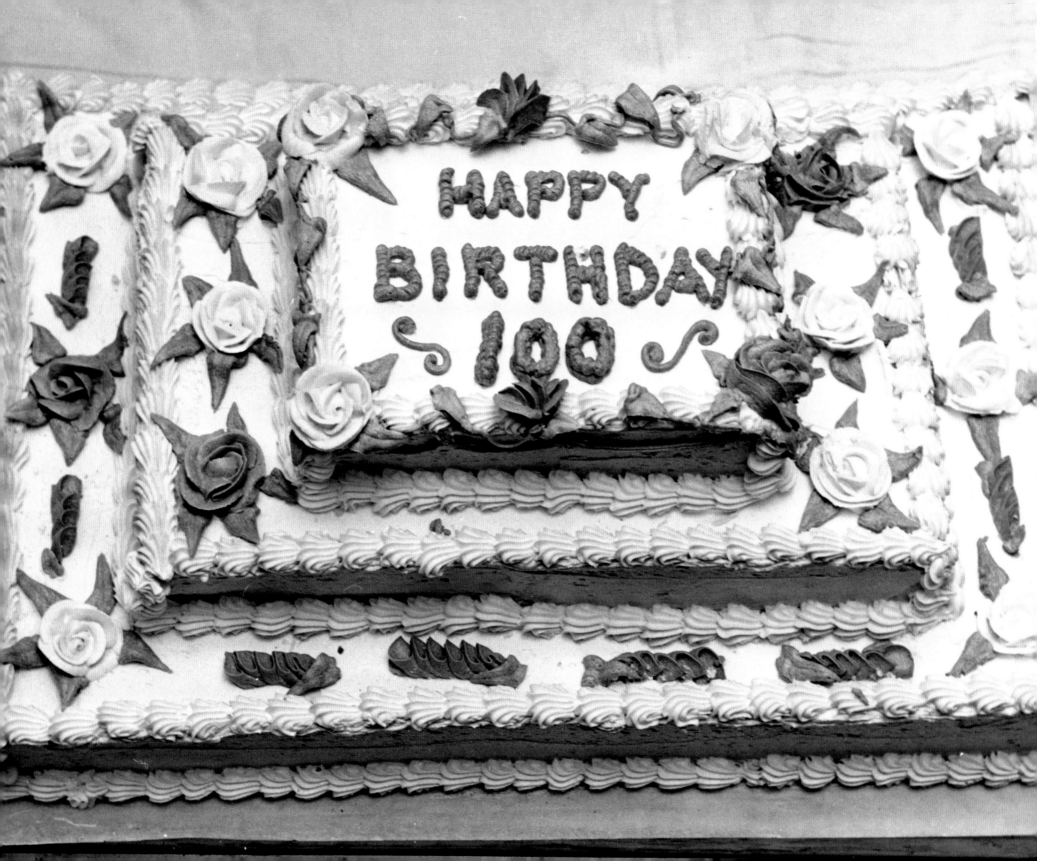

Centennial Planning

Planning for the one-hundredth anniversary of St. Louis State Hospital started early. The Centennial Committee was formed in November 1966. Members were chosen by hospital administration for their leadership abilities and interest in history. Part of the committee focused on ways to celebrate, while another group began research to compile a book of the hospital's history.

In June 1968 a survey was published in the *Employees' Bulletin*. The nine questions ranged from a vague speculation on whether the centennial was important to specifics such as how much should be charged for centennial memorabilia like key chains and notepaper. By February 1969 a centennial slogan and design were found on all correspondence. By the beginning of April a year's worth of events had been planned to include the different facets of the hospital community.

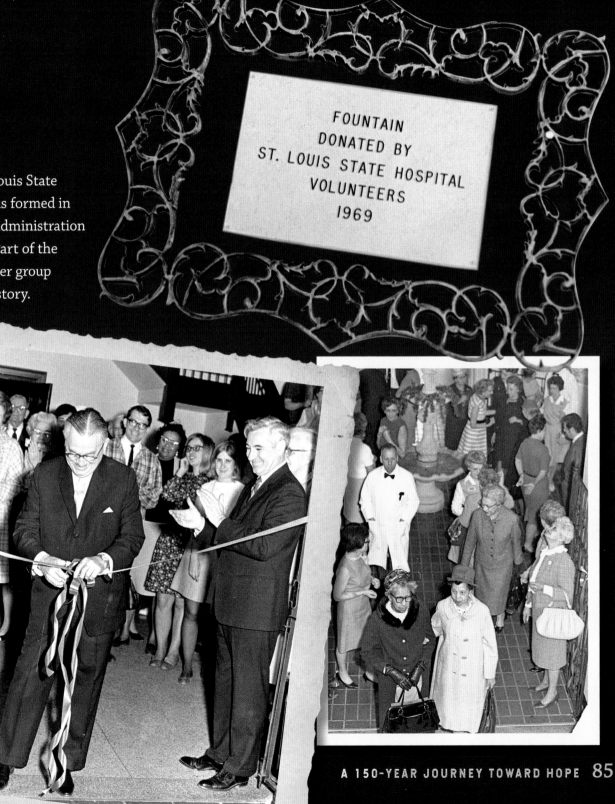

FOUNTAIN
DONATED BY
ST. LOUIS STATE HOSPITAL
VOLUNTEERS
1969

Dr. Kohler cutting the ribbon and opening the Centennial Year, 1969

The Big Day

On April 23, 1969, hospital patients and staff joined the general public to celebrate one hundred years of service. The ceremony began with a rousing number by the Southwest High School band. A Marine Color Guard raised the American flag on the east flagpole and then slowly lowered it to half-mast in honor of President Eisenhower's recent death. A state trooper followed a similar procedure on the west flagpole with the State of Missouri and Centennial flags. A recitation of the Pledge of Allegiance and speech by Superintendent Knowles concluded the ceremony. Dr. Kohler was on hand to cut the ceremonial Centennial ribbon, kicking off the year of celebration and recognition.

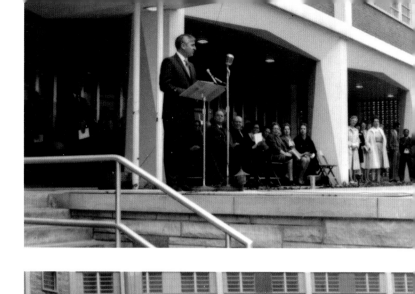

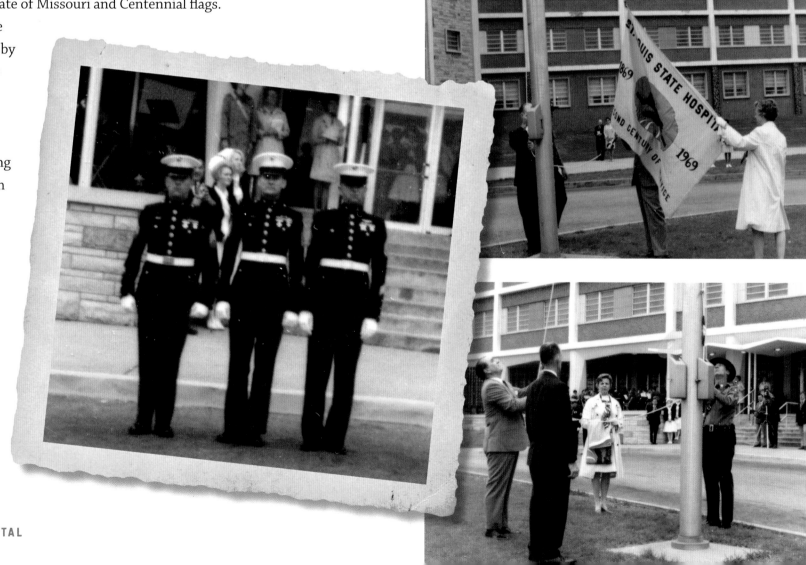

Historic Proclamation

On October 21, 1969, the hospital's centennial year gained its ultimate recognition with a proclamation from the City of St. Louis. That morning Dr. Holden, Dr. Knowles, Dr. Kohler, and Miss Gulmi reunited at City Hall to meet with Mayor A. J. Cervantes. The quartet looked on as Cervantes officially proclaimed November 1969 a month of "Recognition of the Saint Louis State Hospital Centennial." After the signing, the three superintendents posed for a photo representing the hospital's past, present, and future.

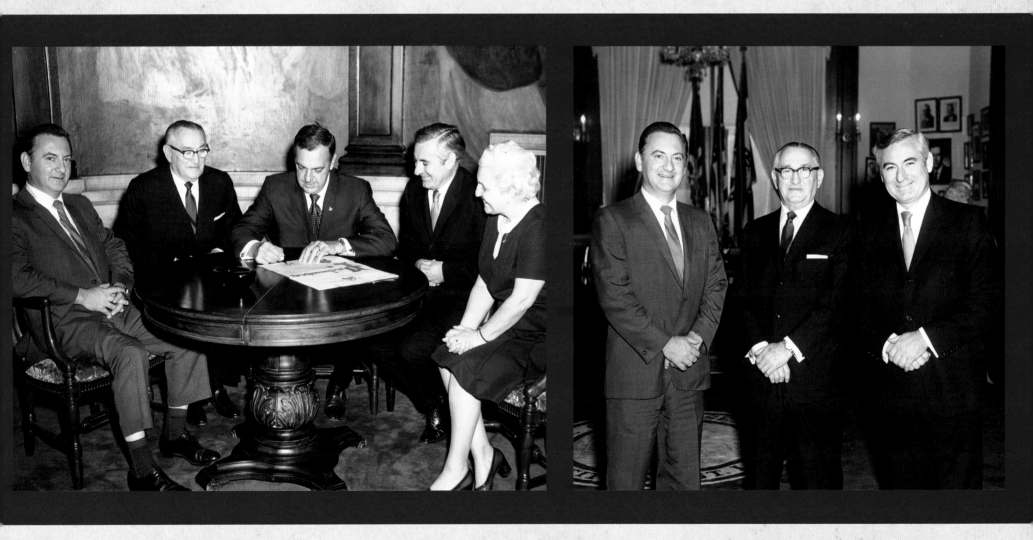

Fall Festival

Even the annual patient carnival followed the centennial theme. The city's early German heritage was honored with a German band and a biergarten serving root beer. A large helium hot air balloon look-alike hovered over the crowd as a tribute to the 1904 World's Fair. The Roaring Twenties were represented by a Charleston contest purporting to be a "challenge to old and young alike!" To showcase the modern age, local radio host Don Miller and his Trafficopter took off and landed throughout the day from the back parking lot, much to the delight of spectators.

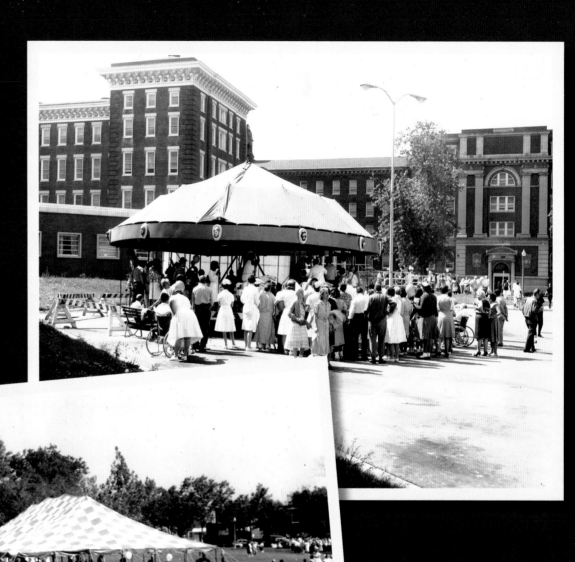

Closing Celebration

The final celebration of the centennial year was held on April 20, 1970. More than four hundred employees, retirees, and members of the public attended a banquet at Ruggeri's Restaurant on the Hill. Tickets to the event included an open bar and a sit-down meal. Dr. Knowles acted as master of ceremonies. Dr. Kohler reminisced on the past, and Dr. Holden outlined the hospital's future.

The evening culminated in the release of the long-awaited history book. *One Hundred Years: The History of St. Louis State Hospital* represented years of research by historian Wilbur Shankland and his committee of assistants. The author, James Dutson, read from the work and held a book signing. Copies were sold for one dollar, with proceeds going to the Auxiliary.

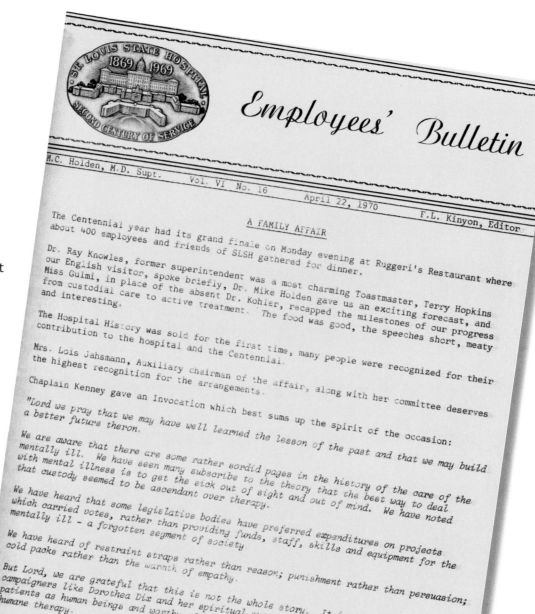

St. Louis State Hospital

Employees' Bulletin

M.C. Holden, M.D. Supt.   Vol. VI No. 16   April 22, 1970   F.L. Kinyon, Editor

A FAMILY AFFAIR

The Centennial year had its grand finale on Monday evening at Ruggeri's Restaurant where about 400 employees and friends of SLSH gathered for dinner.

Dr. Ray Knowles, former superintendent was a most charming Toastmaster, Terry Hopkins our English visitor, spoke briefly, Dr. Mike Holden gave us an exciting forecast, and Miss Gulmi, in place of the absent Dr. Kohler, recapped the milestones of our progress from custodial care to active treatment. The food was good, the speeches short, meaty and interesting.

The Hospital History was sold for the first time, many people were recognized for their contribution to the hospital and the Centennial.

Mrs. Lois Jahsmann, Auxiliary chairman of the affair, along with her committee deserves the highest recognition for the arrangements.

Chaplain Kenney gave an Invocation which best sums up the spirit of the occasion:

"Lord we pray that we may have well learned the lesson of the past and that we may build a better future thereon.

We are aware that there are some rather sordid pages in the history of the care of the mentally ill. We have seen many subscribe to the theory that the best way to deal with mental illness is to get the sick out of sight and out of mind. We have noted that custody seemed to be ascendant over therapy.

We have heard that some legislative bodies have preferred expenditures on projects which carried votes, rather than providing funds, staff, skills and equipment for the mentally ill - a forgotten segment of society.

We have heard of restraint straps rather than reason; punishment rather than persuasion; cold packs rather than the warmth of empathy.

But Lord, we are grateful that this is not the whole story. It is with joy we recall campaigners like Dorothea Dix and her spiritual successors; men and women who have seen patients as human beings and worthy of being treated with dignity, adequate skill and humane therapy.

We are glad that many unsung folk have worked and are now serving in SLSH Complex.

Give them support and encouragement to make this second century one of significant - skillful and humane care.

Help us not be to content with the progress we have made - but to grow in service.

AMEN"

One Hundred Years: The History of St. Louis State Hospital

In early 1967 the hospital Auxiliary decided to fund a commemorative history book. Local historian Dr. Wilbur Shankland was brought in to lend his expertise and research abilities. He quickly assigned willing members to scour the archives of libraries and government offices in St. Louis and Jefferson City. James Dutson, *Globe-Democrat* reporter and, conveniently, a good friend of Dr. Knowles, agreed to write the book.

The final product was released at the closing centennial event held in 1970. Coming in at twenty pages, the book presented an uneven history of the hospital, as well as tangentially related events. Of the photos used, only five were of the hospital and its personnel. That said, whether due to its importance or its one-dollar price tag, it appeared to be popular with employees.

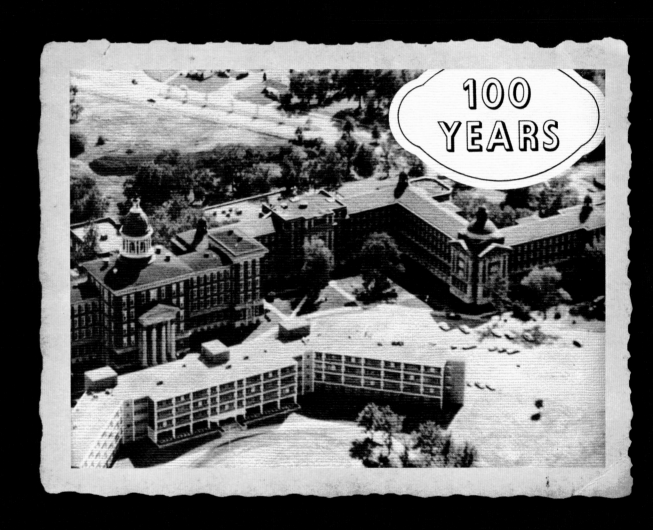

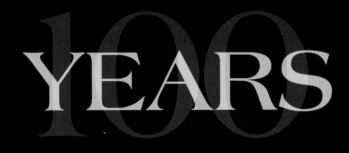

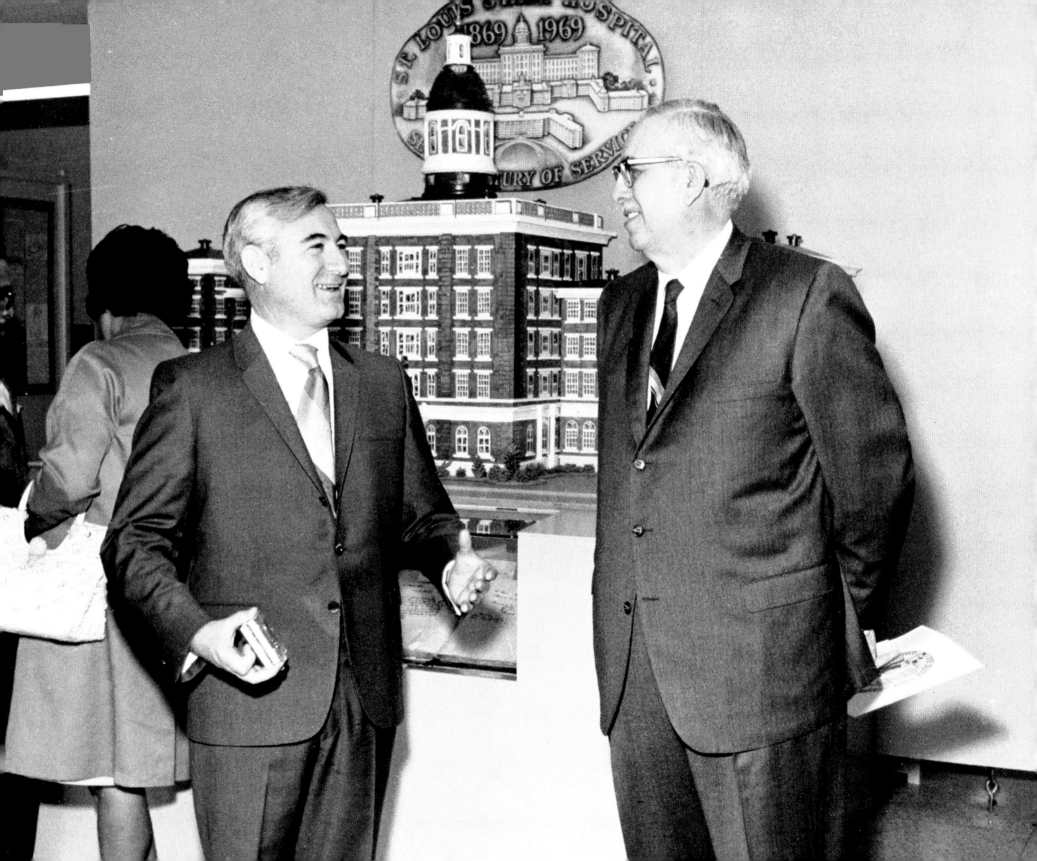

Switchboard Struggles

By 1972 the inpatient population was finally on the decline. However, an increase in research projects, incoming interns, and the various campus clinics kept the three switchboard operators busy throughout the day. In an effort to keep the lines free, pleas from the switchboard were published in almost every issue of the *Bulletin*.

To give readers a taste of life on the switchboard, an operator submitted the following conversations.

Caller: May I speak to Mrs. Jones?
Operator: Do you know what she does here?
Caller: Yes, she is a psychopathic aide.
Operator: Thank you.

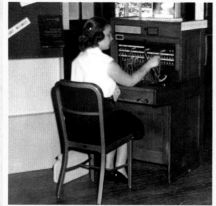

Caller: May I speak to Mrs. Jones on 3C?
Operator: Is she an RN?
Caller: No, operator, she's an American.
Operator: Thank you.

Inside Caller: How do I get an outside line on this phone, operator?
Operator: What phone are you using, sir?
Caller: That's for you to find out, operator.
Operator: Then you'll have to find the way to get an outside line, sir.
Caller: Touché, operator.
Operator: Touché, sir.

Operator: Missouri Institute of Psychiatry (hurriedly).
Caller: Operator, would you please say that again?
Operator: Missouri Institute of Psychiatry (slower).
Caller: You said that so pretty, but I didn't understand a word you said.
Operator: Thank you, I'll slow it down from now on.

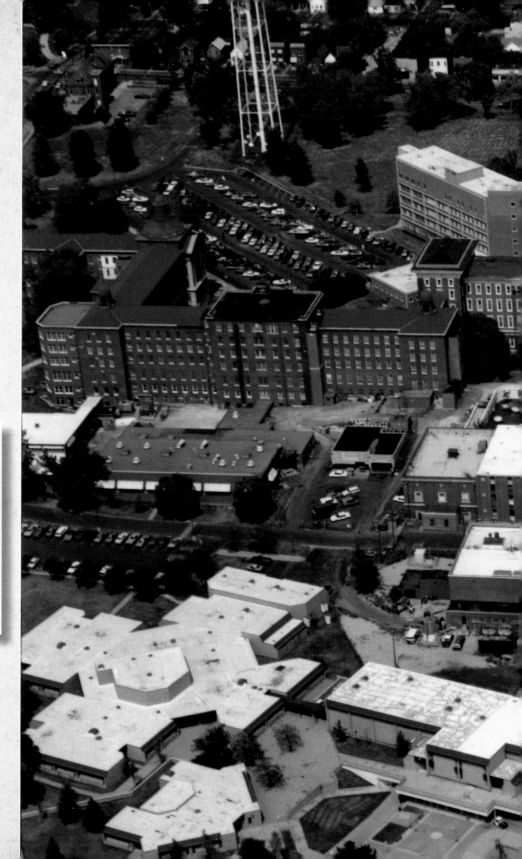

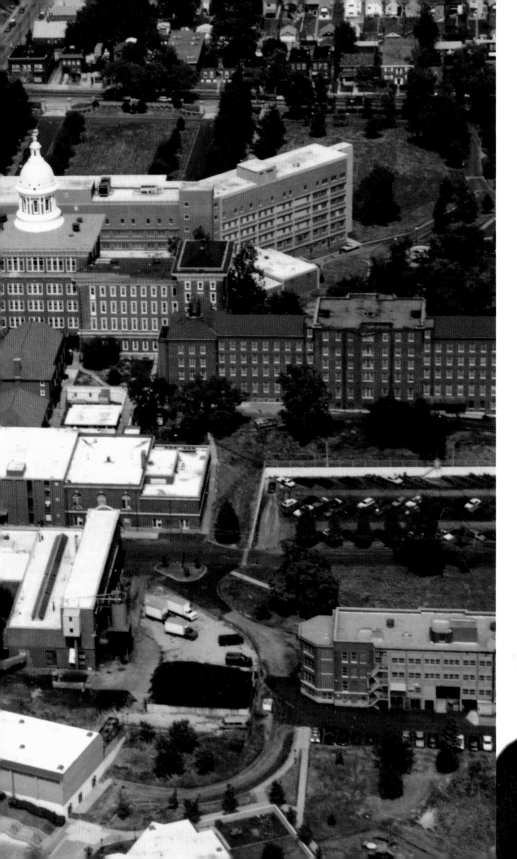

Youth Center Opens

Despite its success, Special School No. 2 fizzled sometime in the 1930s. After several years of trying to provide services to the young population, the administration at last developed programming for youth. Located at various places on campus, the Youth Center provided special education and vocational rehabilitation services. As in the 1920s, most of the focus was on useful life skills. To this end, a fully functioning garage was built to train auto mechanics. Staff were even allowed to drop off their vehicles for free oil changes, tire rotations, and simple maintenance.

In 1976 the state funded the construction of a separate complex on the back grounds dedicated solely to youth. Considered state of the art, the campus consisted of several single-story buildings containing classrooms, living areas, and an indoor pool. By 1981 it was officially known as Hawthorn Children's Psychiatric Hospital.

Unfortunately, by the mid-1980s it was clear that no matter how attractive, the Hawthorn buildings simply were not childproof. Patients would make their escape through fences and climb through the air ducts to freedom. Eventually, a more secure facility would be built off campus and the old Hawthorn sold to a charter school.

Saying Goodbye

The decision to downsize the campus buildings was a blow to employees and patients alike. For all of their problems, the old buildings were beloved and familiar. As a way to say goodbye, as well as to document their existence, extensive work went into photographing the empty wards, corridors, and demolition.

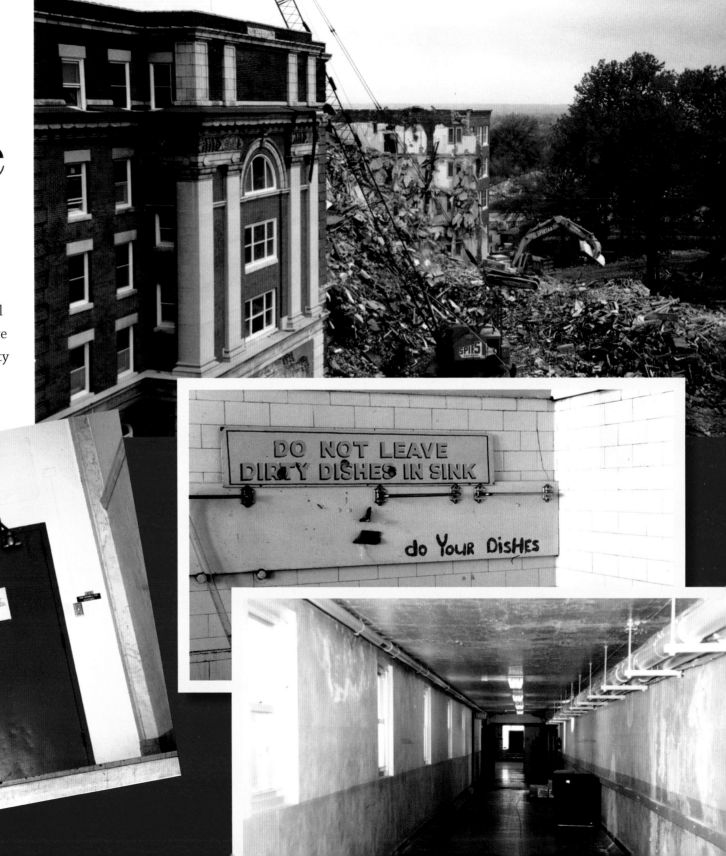

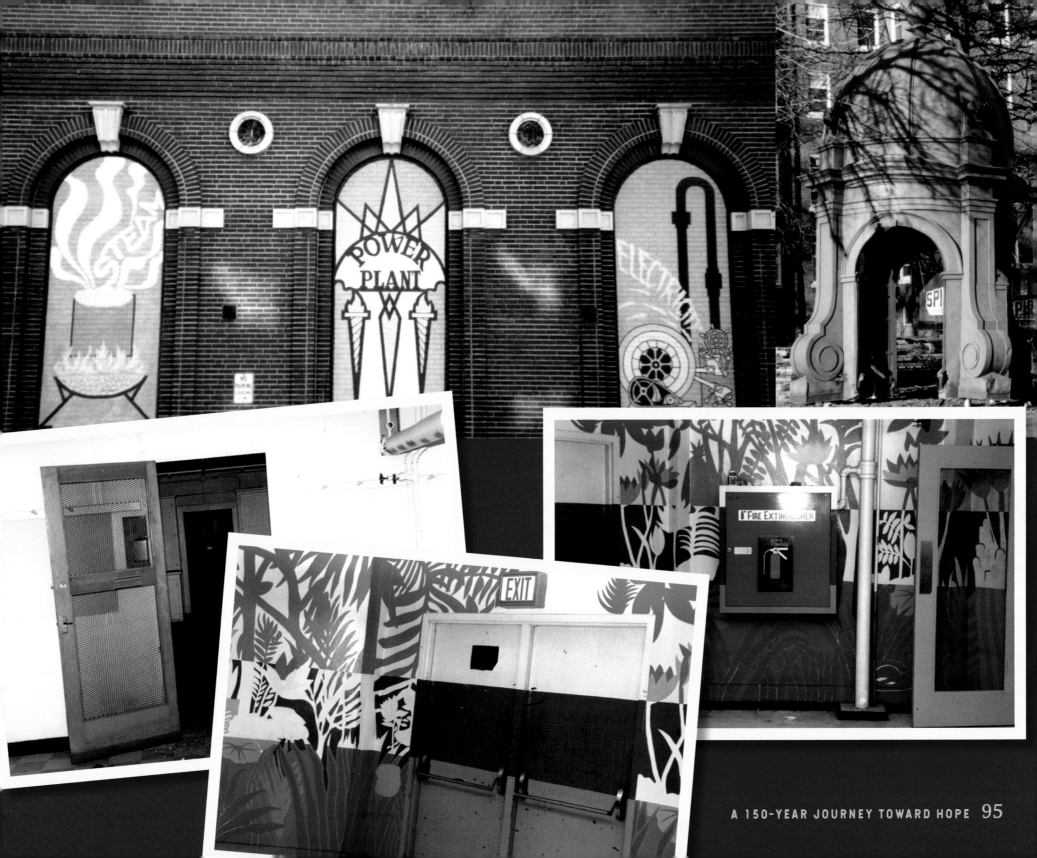

Dr. Fujita's Morale

The financial crisis of the 1980s hit the hospital hard. Layoffs, mandatory days without pay, and hiring freezes left morale at an all-time low. Meanwhile, policies and regulations on a state and federal level were limiting activities. In an attempt to liven spirits, Dr. Fujita instituted what would become his annual Christmas shindig. The event highlighted employee talent, and planning began as early as September. Groups and individuals performed musical numbers as well as skits. Dr. Fujita also took part, showing off his talents and letting his staff know he cared.

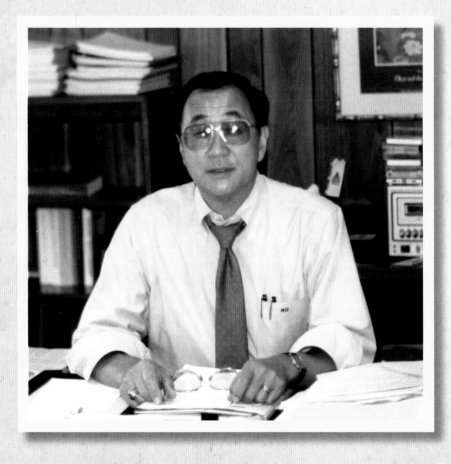

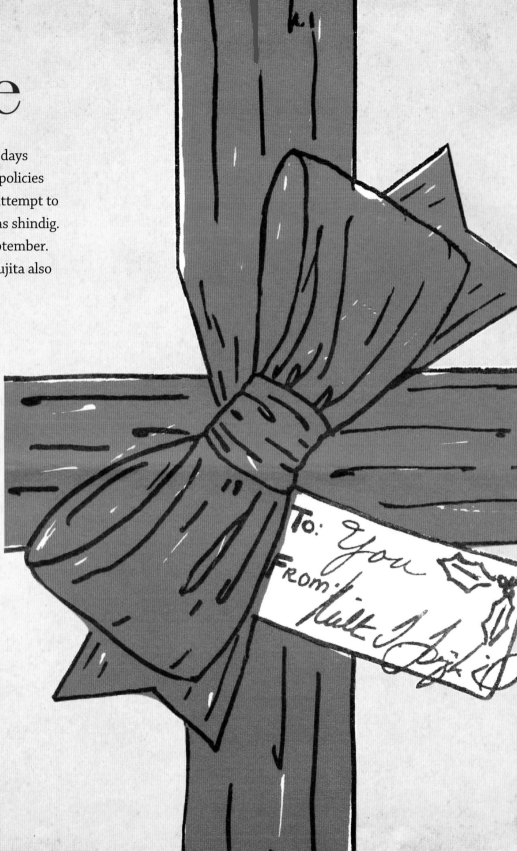

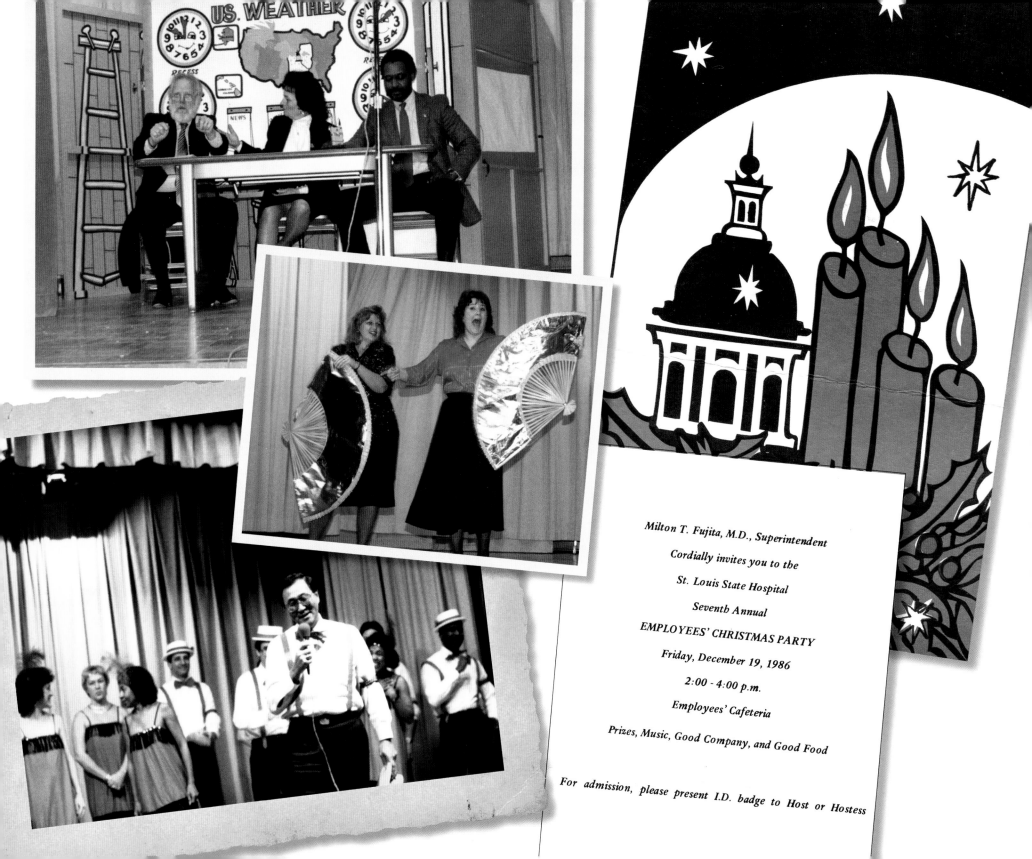

Milton T. Fujita, M.D., Superintendent

Cordially invites you to the

St. Louis State Hospital

Seventh Annual

EMPLOYEES' CHRISTMAS PARTY

Friday, December 19, 1986

2:00 - 4:00 p.m.

Employees' Cafeteria

Prizes, Music, Good Company, and Good Food

For admission, please present I.D. badge to Host or Hostess

Fireworks

During the late 1970s and early 1980s, St. Louis State Hospital went all out celebrating patriotism. To cap off the annual picnic, a giant fireworks display was launched from the front lawn. Touted as the largest in South City, the display contained more than seven hundred types of fireworks synchronized with music. Patients, staff, and the community watched the show, which could be seen from miles away.

Giant Fireworks Display

A gigantic fireworks display will be held on St. Louis State Hospital grounds at 8:00 p.m. Thursday, July 3. More than 700 fireworks will be ignited, featuring aerial displays visible up to 30 miles. In the event of rain, the fireworks display will be held the following evening. The fireworks will be provided by The S.H.I.P Program.

October-November 1980

OUTLOOK

St. Louis State Hospital Complex

5400 Arsenal Street
St. Louis, Missouri 63139

Celebrating Independence Day

St. Louis State Hospital entered into the ranks of big-time pyrotechnics with a spectacular fireworks display on the evening of July 3 as part of an Independence Day celebration, held on the front grounds of the hospital, for the enjoyment of patients, their families and friends, as well as the neighboring community. About 2,000 persons attended the celebration which was sponsored by S.H.I.P. (State Hospital Industrial Program). In addition to the fireworks display, the celebration included live band music, refreshments, appearances by various state dignitaries and presentations of awards to The St. Louis City Fire Department. A special recognition to fire-fighter John Turin, of Hook and Ladder Company 10, was made for his successful life-saving rescue of a patient in May. Mr. Turin's award was presented by Mr. Walter Sloan, president of the hospital's Patient Advocacy Group, on behalf of that organization (top left). Starting at dusk, a professional pyrotechnician went about his task as 733 rockets and flares were launched from buried tubes, exploding in the air and throwing dazzling sparks and whistles on their journey back to earth. The pyrotechnician created a safe and beautiful show that thoroughly entertained the crowd. As the ear-popping giant firework finale ended, Gene Burbes, director of S.H.I.P., yelled over the microphone: "That concludes our 1980 Independence Day celebration . . . did you like the fireworks? Wait 'til next year!" The crowd gave its hearty approval. Discussing the celebration, Mr. Burbes said, "We hope this event will be considered as a positive endeavor of the hospital to bring itself into a closer acquaintanceship with the community.

206 Receive CPR Training

A total of 206 nurses and other hospital personnel at St. Louis State Hospital have undergone extensive in-service training in Cardio Pulmonary Resuscitation (CPR) at the hospital in recent months. The training includes three hours of instruction, using the standards of the American Heart Association.

Persons training in CPR can come to the aid of victims of a heart attack, electrical shock, drowning, suffocation, choking, head injury or sudden death.

CPR consists of opening and maintaining an open airway, providing artificial ventilation by means of mouth-to-mouth breathing and providing artificial circulation by means of external chest compressions, according to Sarah Carr, R.N., primary instructor of the State Hospital program. The training is designed to enable State Hospital personnel to provide emergency assistance through standardized treatment procedures, possibly preventing premature death, Ms. Carr said.

According to the St. Louis Heart Association, 18,000 persons, in the St. Louis area, were trained in basic life-support CPR last year.

125th Anniversary

April 23, 1994, marked the 125th anniversary of the hospital complex. As with the centennial, planning began in advance. A history committee was formed and held monthly meetings. Staff and patients contributed ideas for events and commemorations. One early hope was for a sequel to the 1969 St. Louis State Hospital history book, but the recent budgetary problems made it impossible to obtain the necessary funding. In lieu of a written record, the committee ultimately decided on a time capsule.

ST. LOUIS
STATE
HOSPITAL

125TH ANNIVERSARY
1869·1994

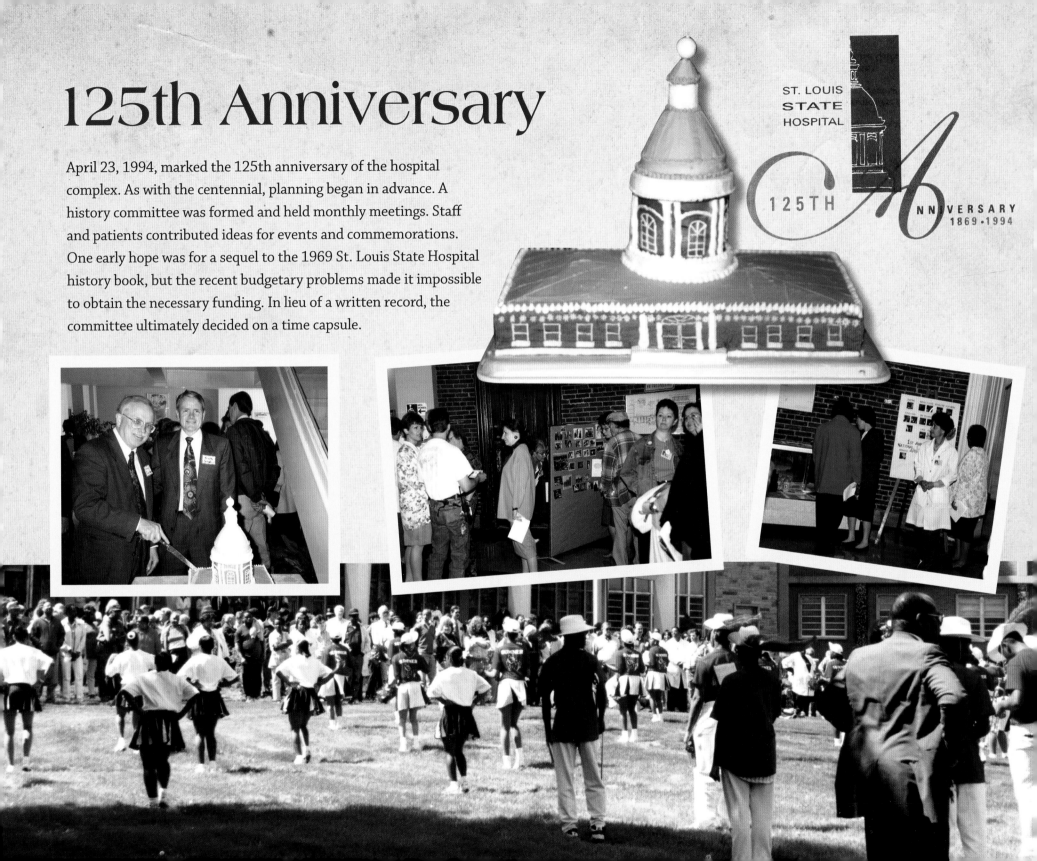

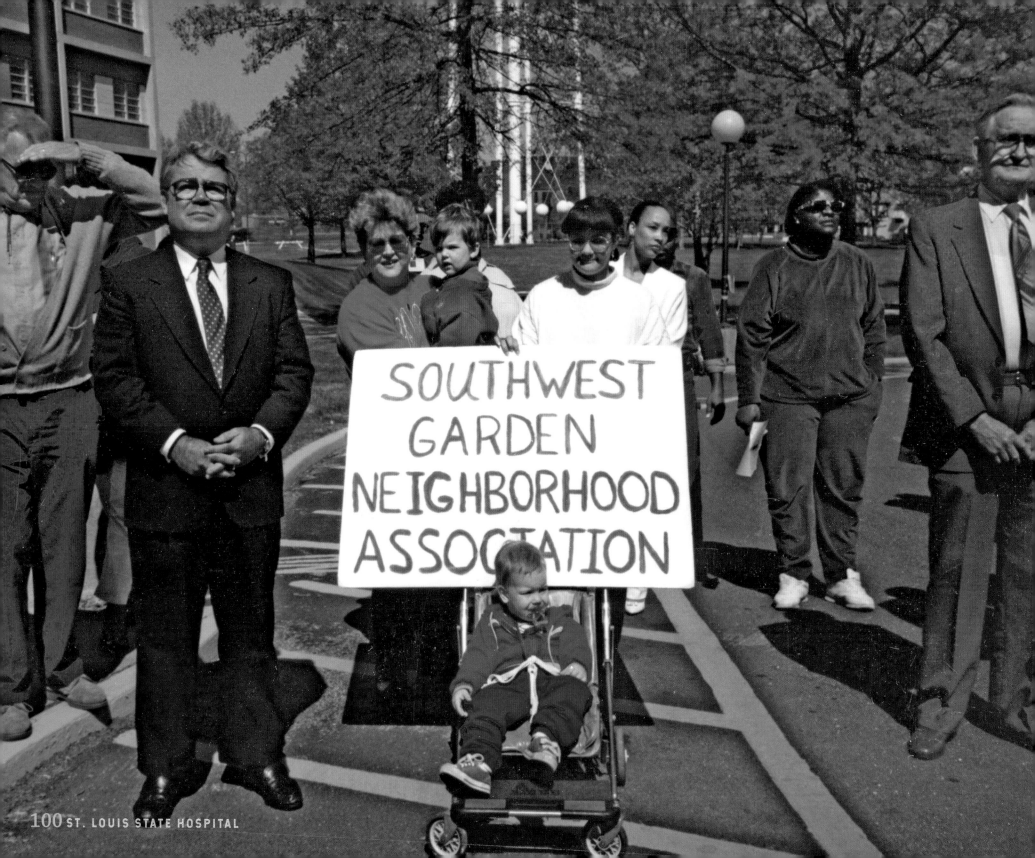

To Be Opened in 2094

The maintenance department got busy crafting the capsule from PVC pipe while the history committee solicited for items to include. The 125th anniversary logo was painted on the outside in the hospital green and white. On April 23 members of the Southwest Garden Neighborhood Association, retirees, patients, and staff gathered on the front lawn. Former superintendents Dr. Knowles and Dr. Hofstatter, both of rather advanced years, ceremoniously broke ground before letting younger folks finish the job.

The history committee decided on the contents of the time capsule based on the mission of the hospital and the outlook for mental illness in the 1990s. The majority of the contents ended up being program manuals, policies, and various forms of paperwork. More tangible items included a button, sticker, and mug. The contents list also mentions "two reindeer" and an "icicle," with no explanation.

Unlike the ill-fated time capsules of 1864 and 1970, this one's location was well marked on the front lawn by a large rock. A bronze plaque affixed to the rock explains what it guards and gives clear instructions that the capsule is to only be opened in one hundred years.

Dr. Knowles and Dr. Hofstatter breaking ground, 1994

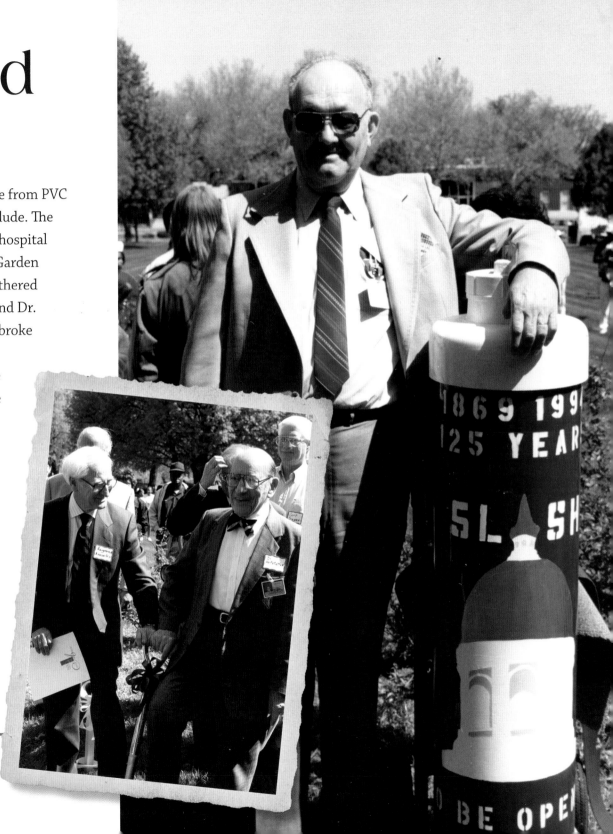

New Beginnings Picnic

To get staff and patients excited about the new building projects, a special picnic was held. Food, music, and games gave everyone a break from the stress of moving. The dunk tank and pie-throwing booth allowed employees to let off a little steam at the good sports who volunteered to take one for the team.

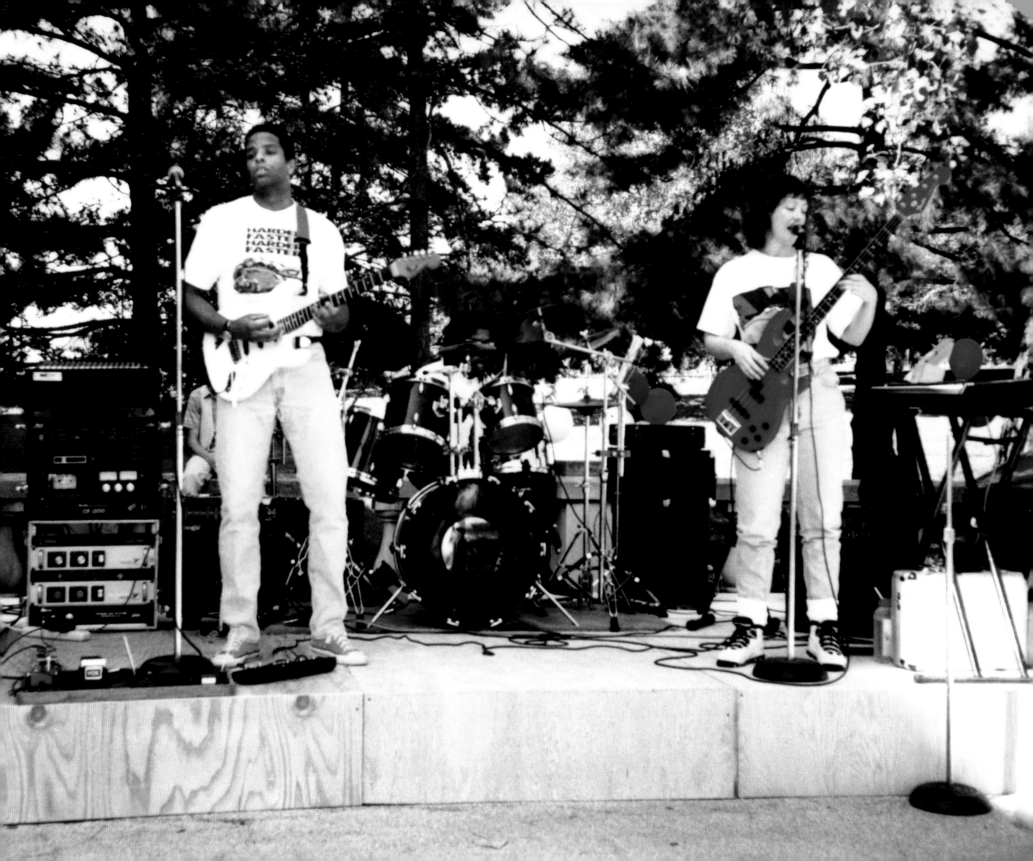

Demolition and Looking Forward

The significant downsizing of the late 1980s and early 1990s left the campus a shell of its former self. To better accommodate the new patient and staff numbers, construction began on a smaller and more secure building. Located on the corner of the campus once occupied by the Employees' Building, the new hospital featured a simple design surrounding a courtyard. Four wings would hold twenty-five patients each, while freestanding cottages could accommodate eight to ten people. Meanwhile, the crumbling Kohler building, vacant west wing, and old water tower would come down. After several years of steady construction, the new building was dedicated on October 21, 1997. In honor of the occasion, a contest was held to rename the facility. Ultimately, St. Louis Psychiatric Rehabilitation Center was chosen to highlight the new focus on recovery.

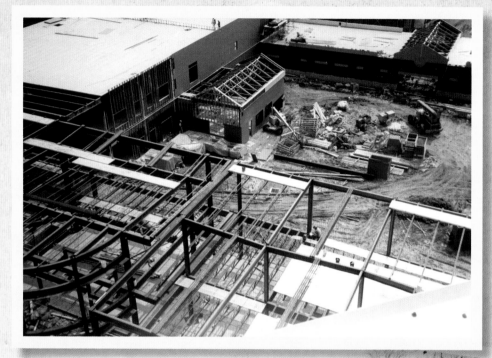

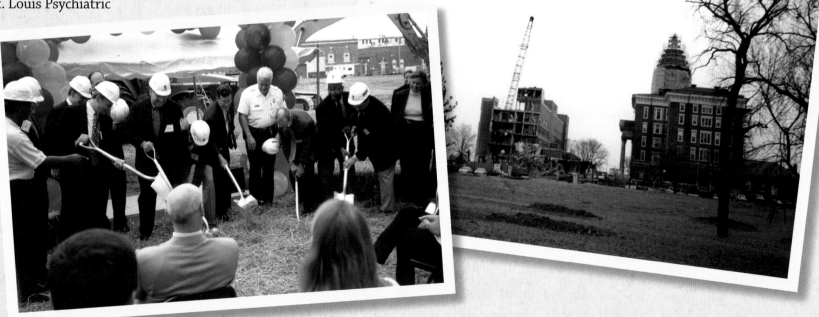

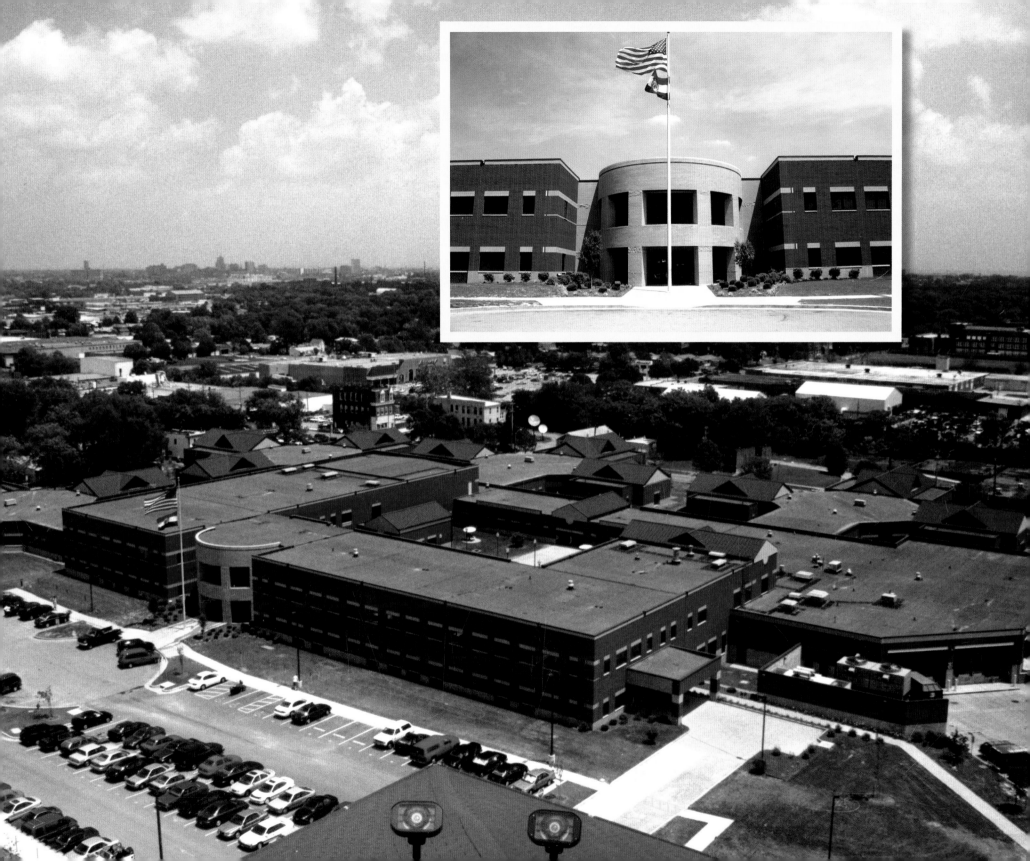

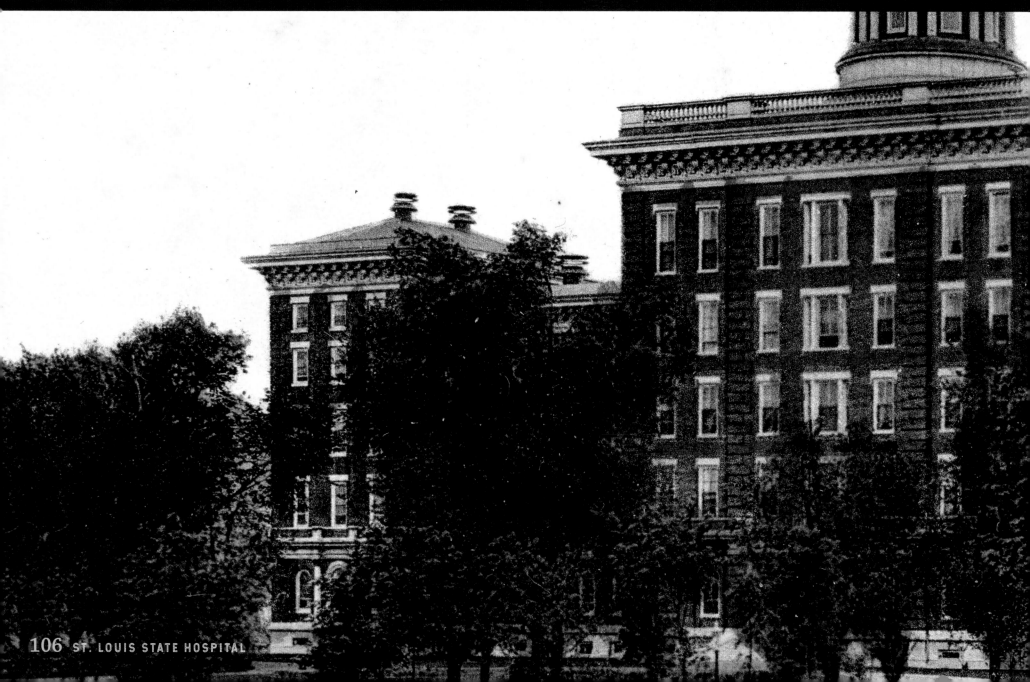

1905

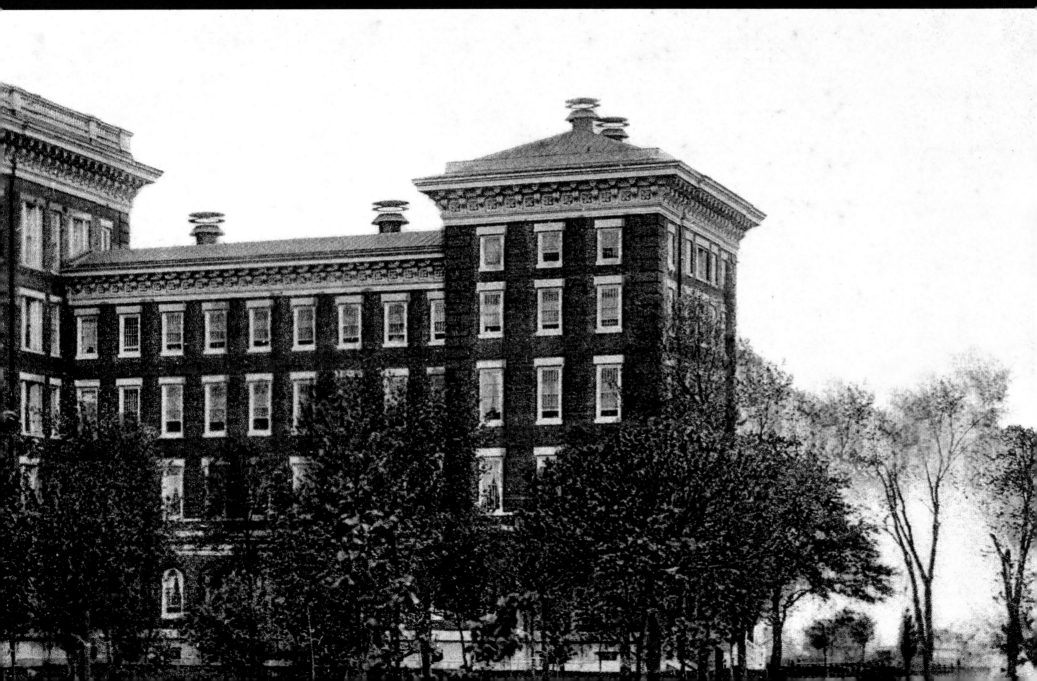

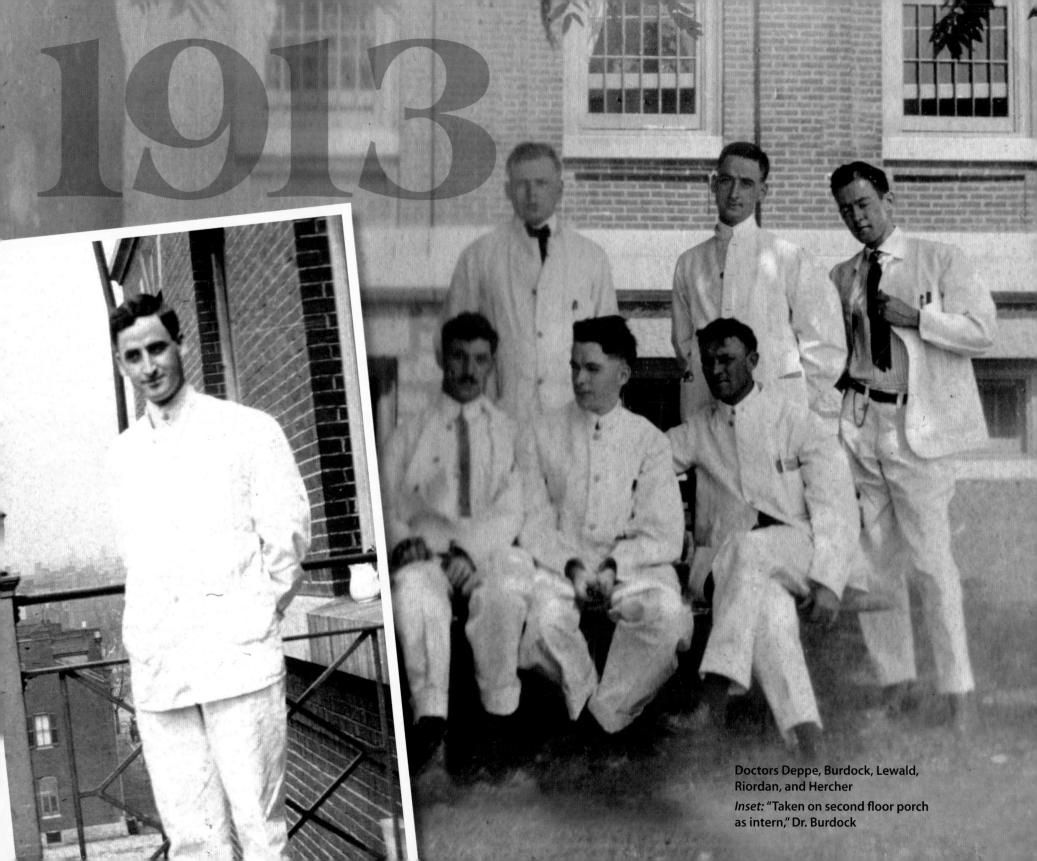

1913

Doctors Deppe, Burdock, Lewald, Riordan, and Hercher

Inset: "Taken on second floor porch as intern," Dr. Burdock

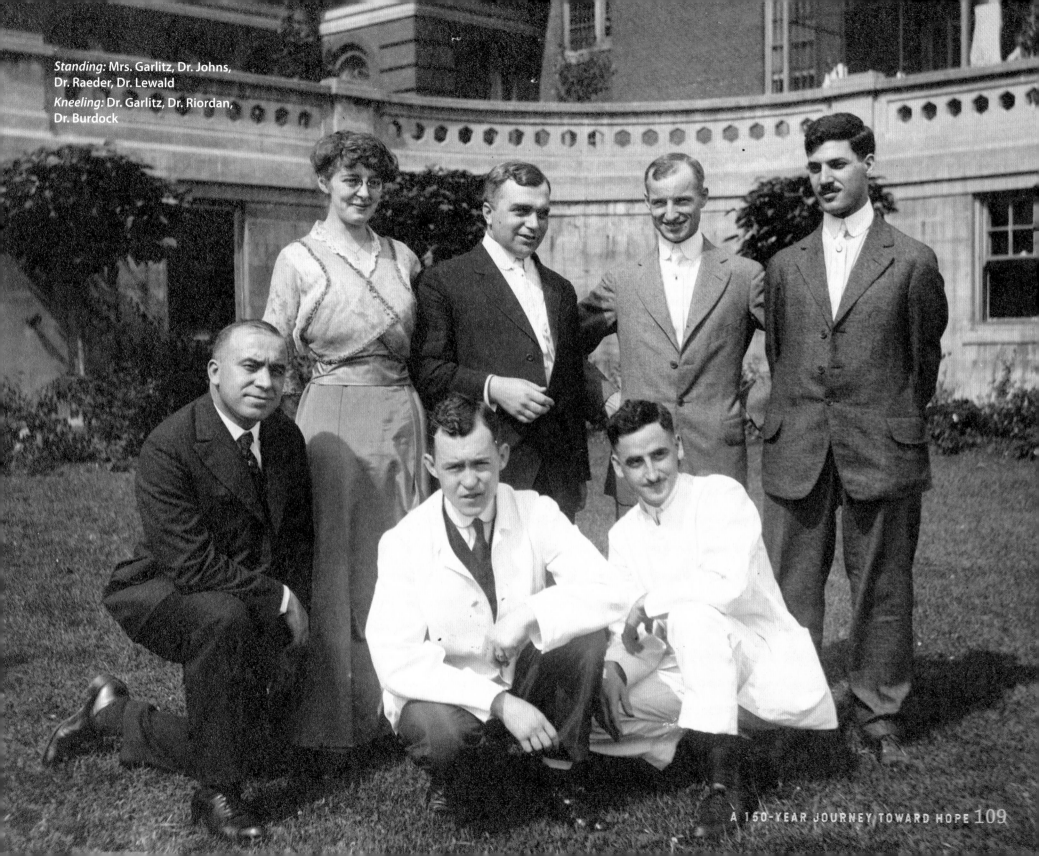

Standing: Mrs. Garlitz, Dr. Johns, Dr. Raeder, Dr. Lewald
Kneeling: Dr. Garlitz, Dr. Riordan, Dr. Burdock

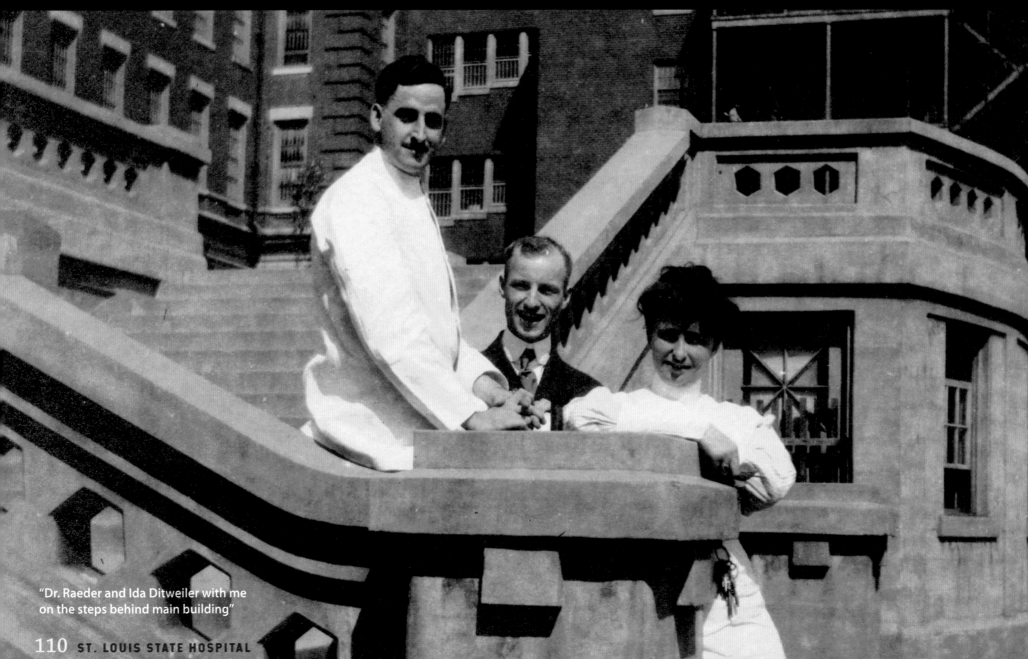

1915

"Dr. Raeder and Ida Ditweiler with me on the steps behind main building"

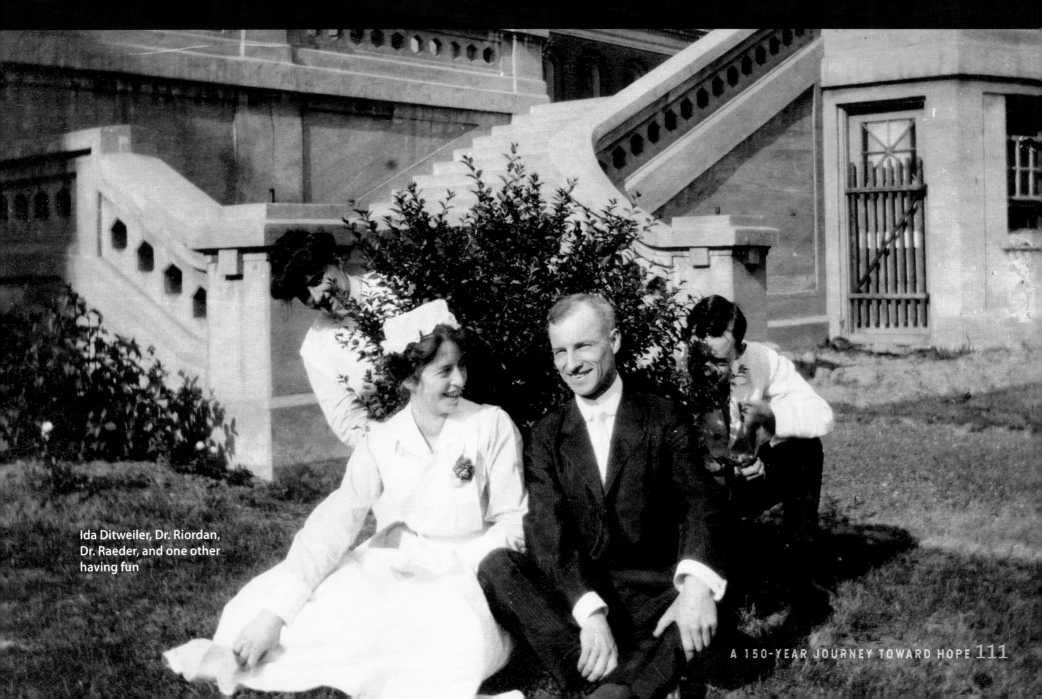

Doctors, Attendants, and Patients

Ida Ditweiler, Dr. Riordan, Dr. Raeder, and one other having fun

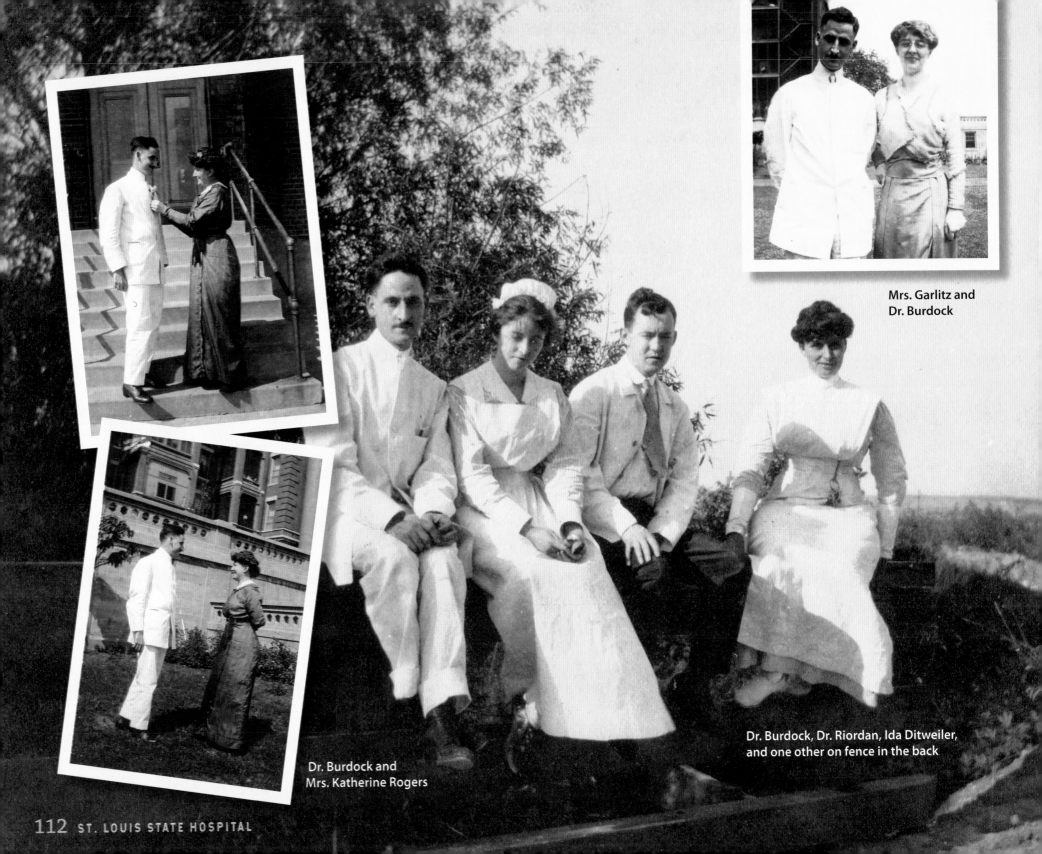

Mrs. Garlitz and
Dr. Burdock

Dr. Burdock, Dr. Riordan, Ida Ditweiler,
and one other on fence in the back

Dr. Burdock and
Mrs. Katherine Rogers

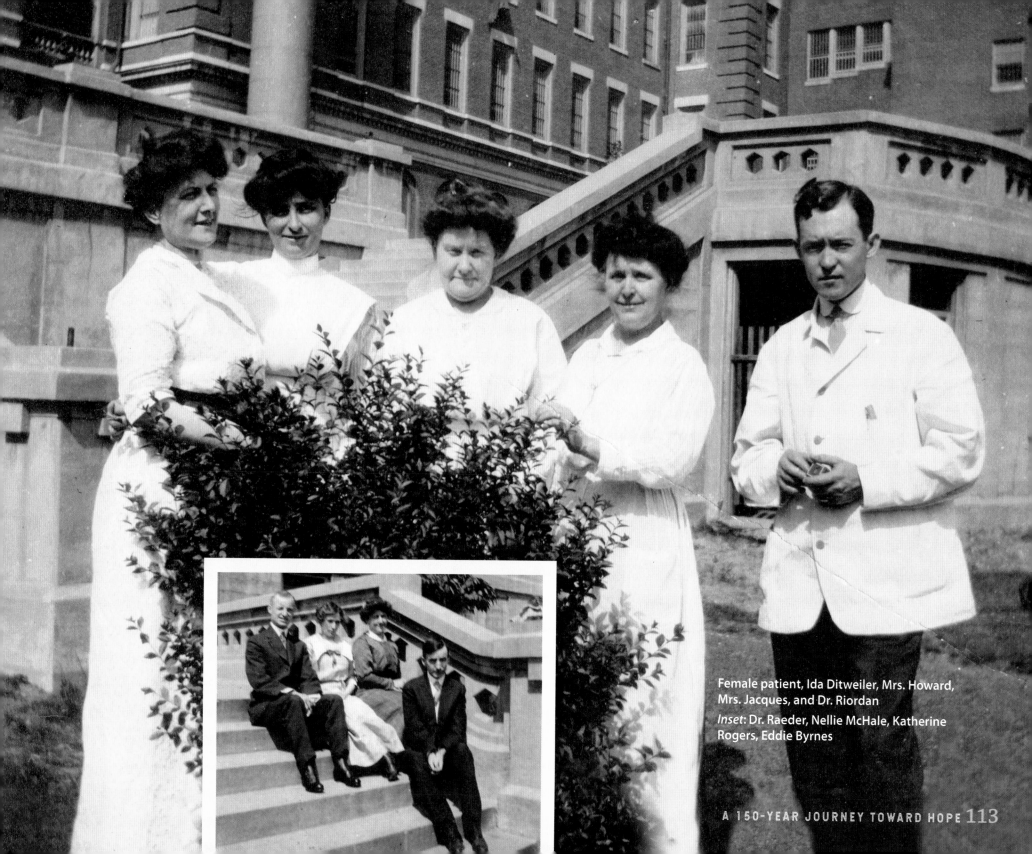

Female patient, Ida Ditweiler, Mrs. Howard, Mrs. Jacques, and Dr. Riordan

Inset: Dr. Raeder, Nellie McHale, Katherine Rogers, Eddie Byrnes

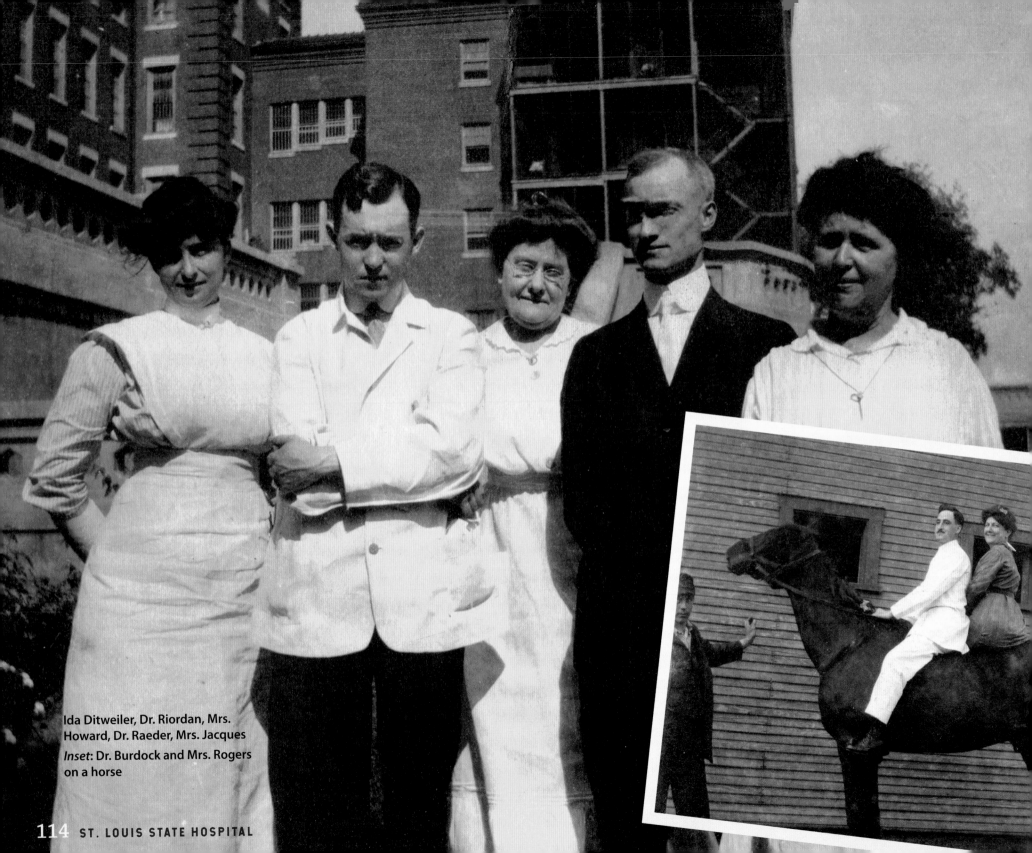

Ida Ditweiler, Dr. Riordan, Mrs. Howard, Dr. Raeder, Mrs. Jacques

Inset: Dr. Burdock and Mrs. Rogers on a horse

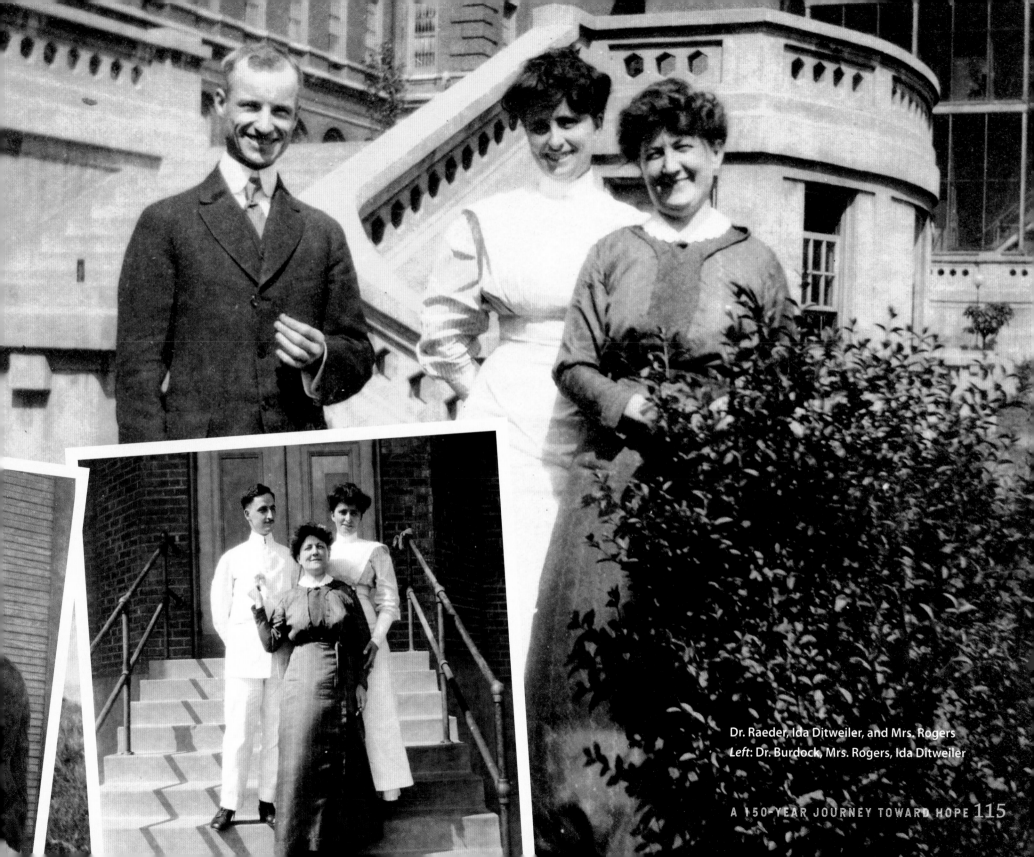

Dr. Raeder, Ida Ditweiler, and Mrs. Rogers
Left: Dr. Burdock, Mrs. Rogers, Ida Ditweiler

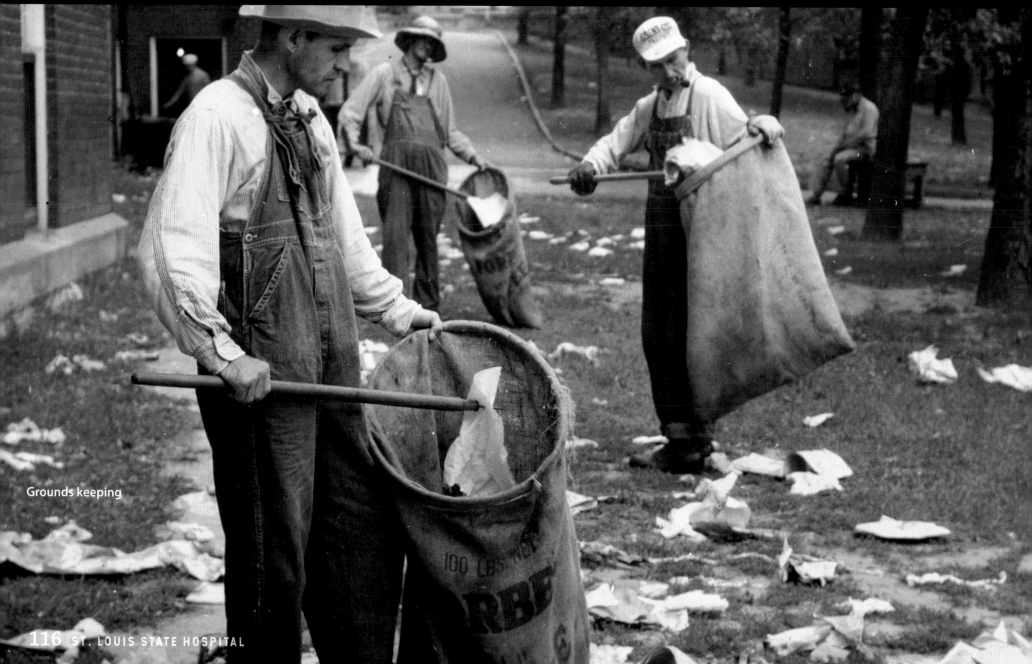

Grounds keeping

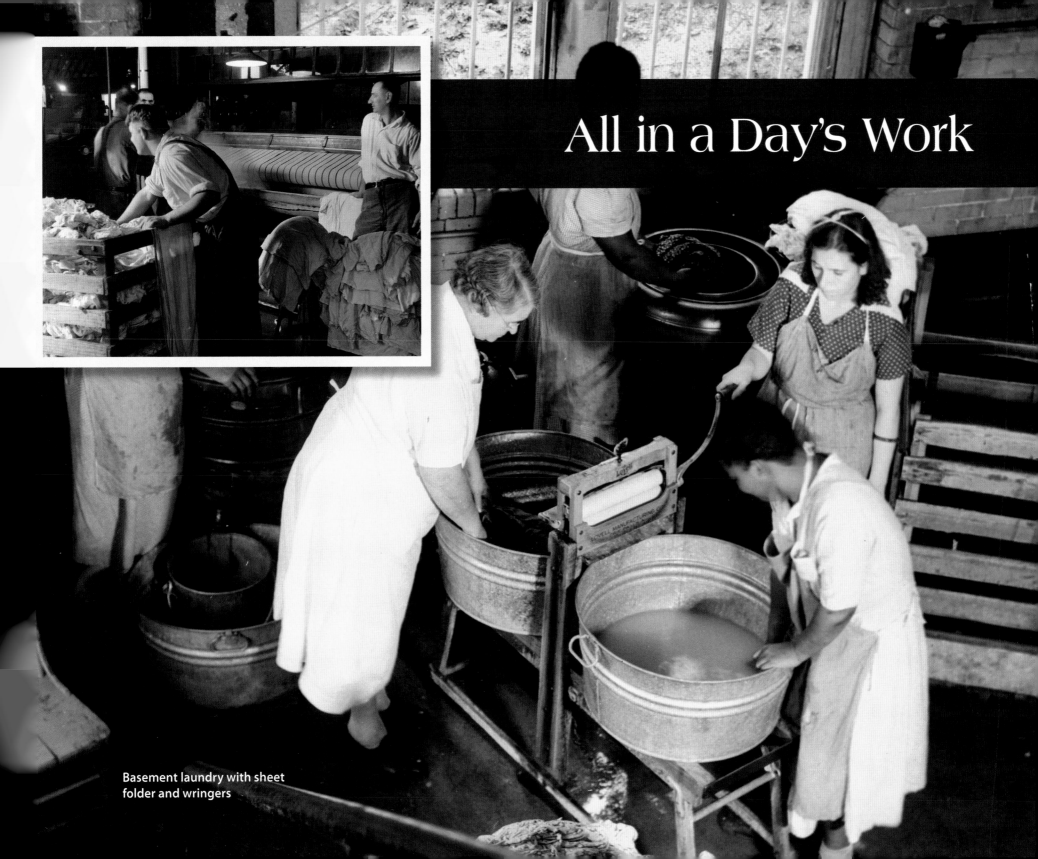

All in a Day's Work

Basement laundry with sheet folder and wringers

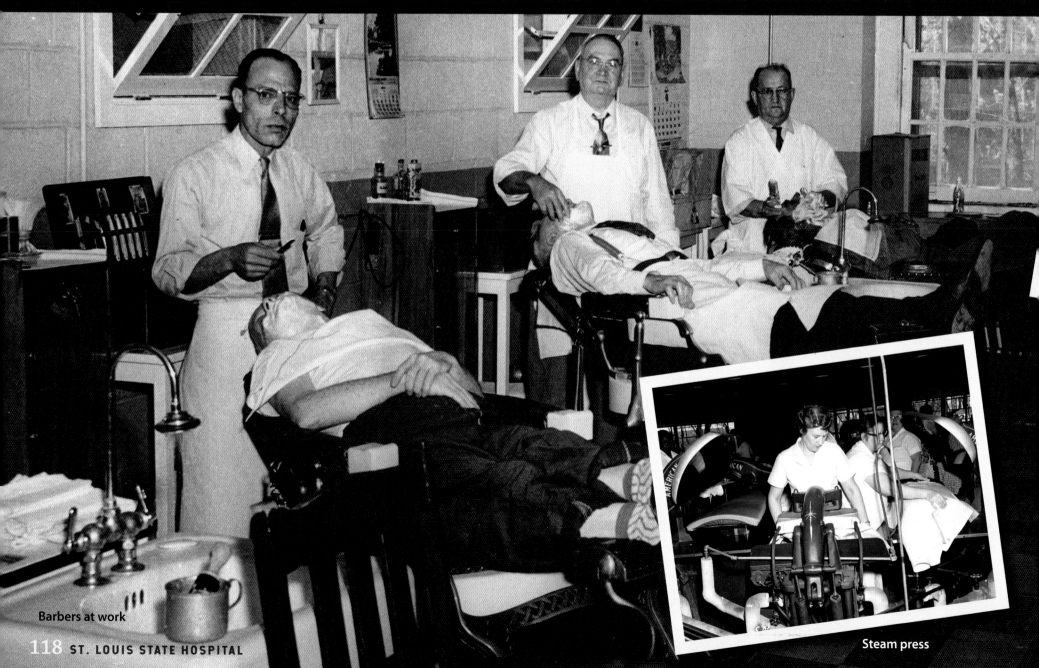

1950

Barbers at work

Steam press

Pot washing

Paul Baroli, Cook 1 and Joe Foster, Food Manager 1

1954

Tile shop

Carpenter shop

1955

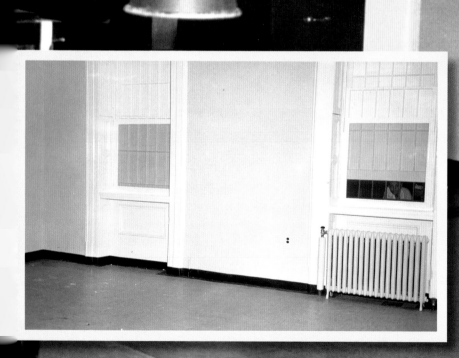

5th Floor Rennovation

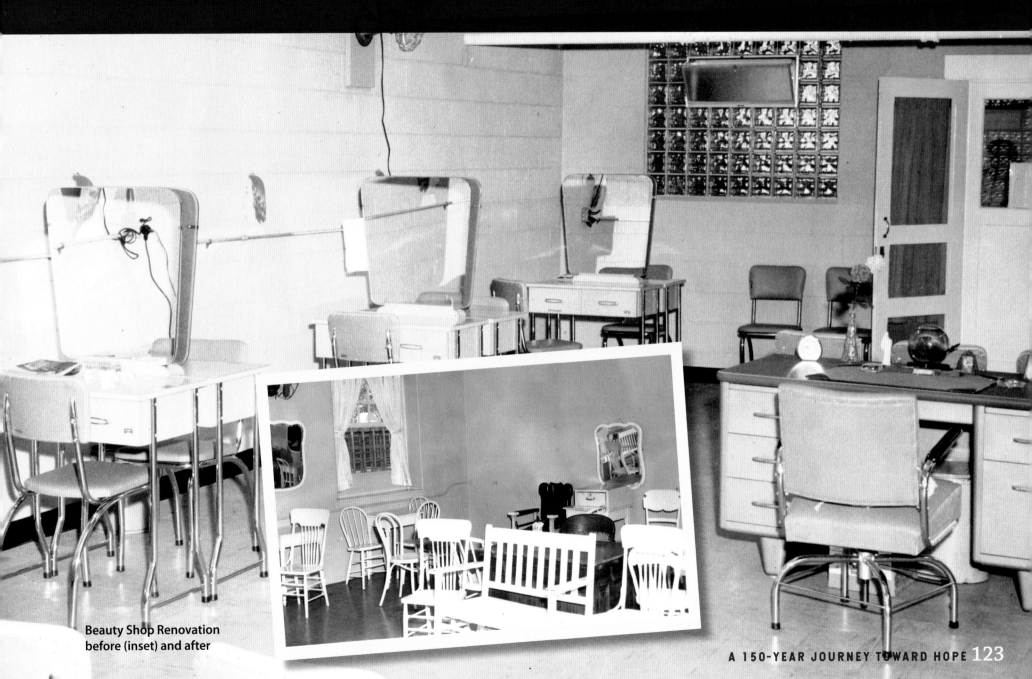

Renovations Before and After

Beauty Shop Renovation
before (inset) and after

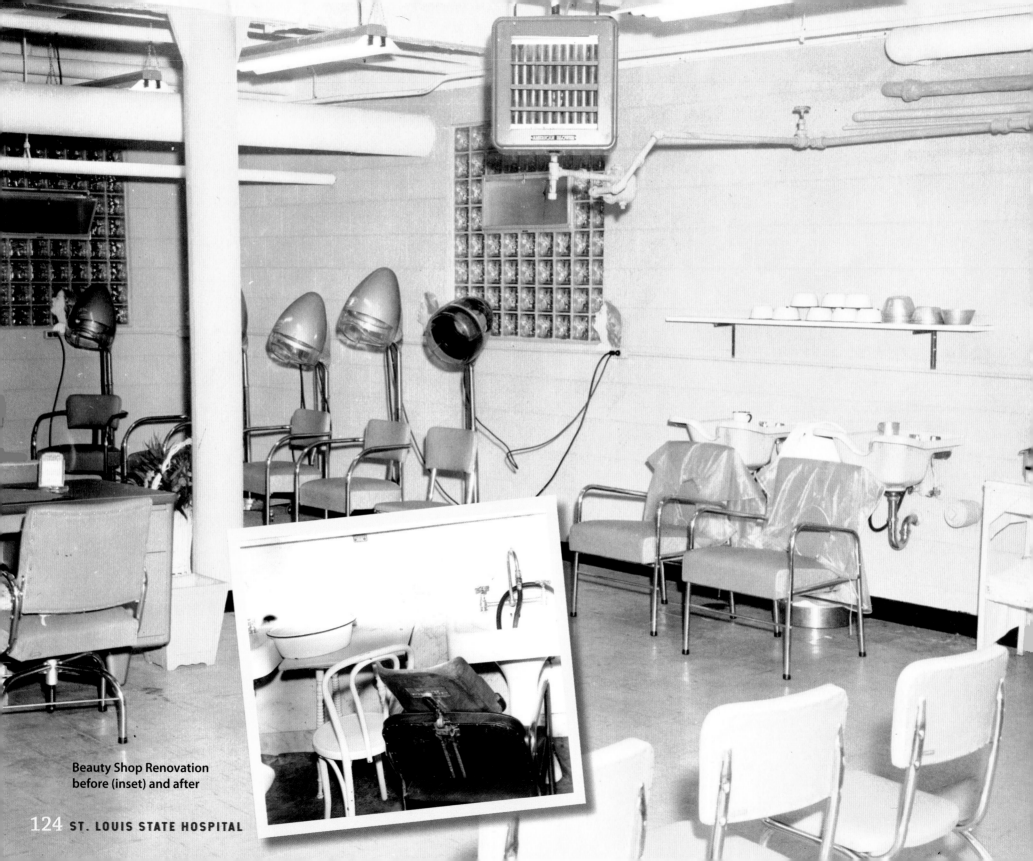

Beauty Shop Renovation
before (inset) and after

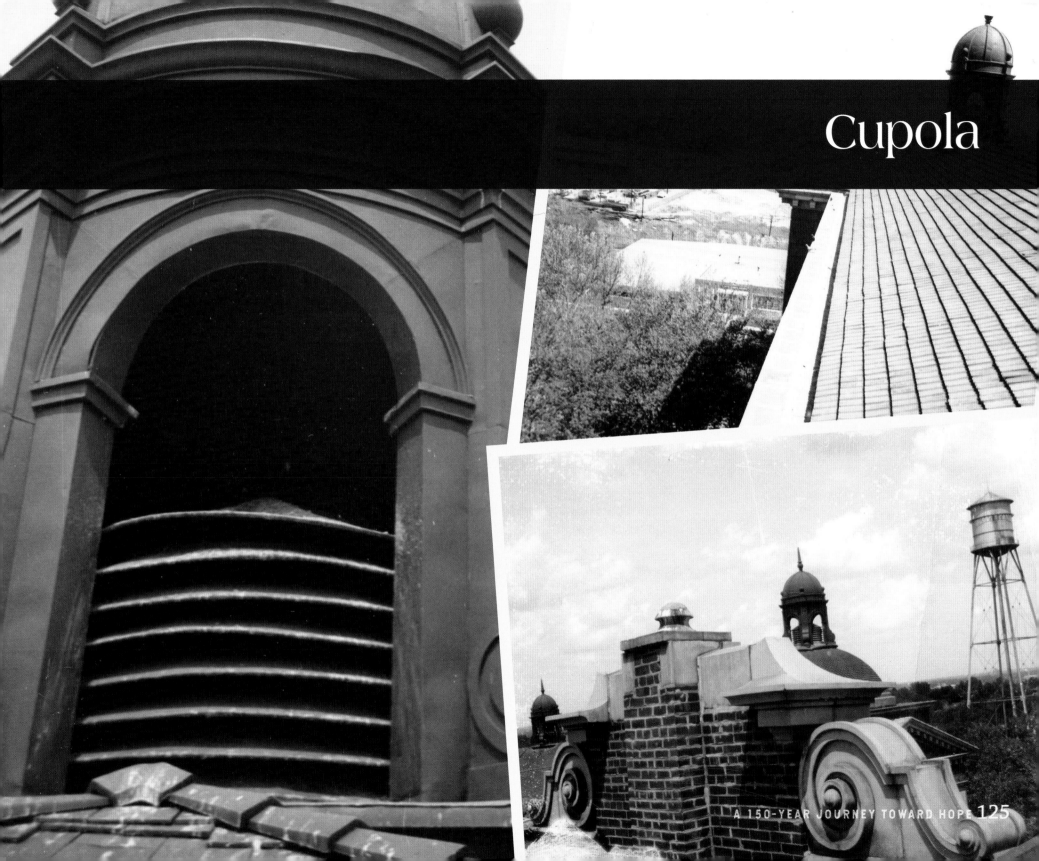

1976

Hook and ladder at the Kohler Building

Inset: Firetruck ladder to top of Kohler Building

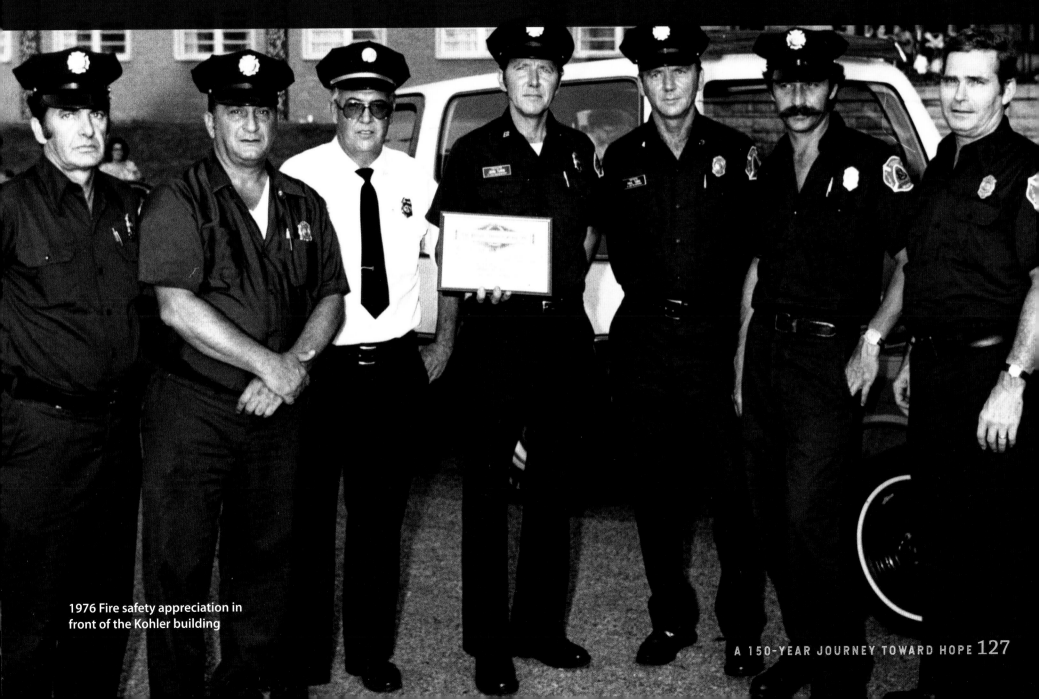

Fire Safety

1976 Fire safety appreciation in front of the Kohler building

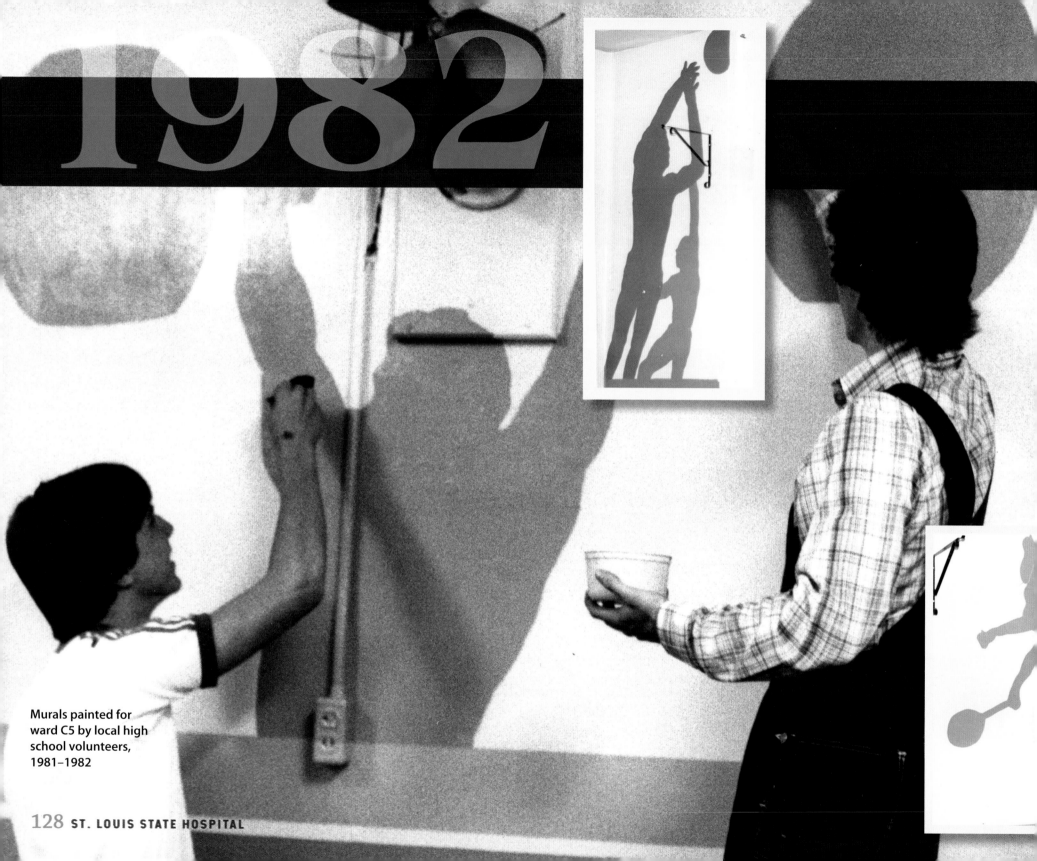

1982

Murals painted for ward C5 by local high school volunteers, 1981–1982

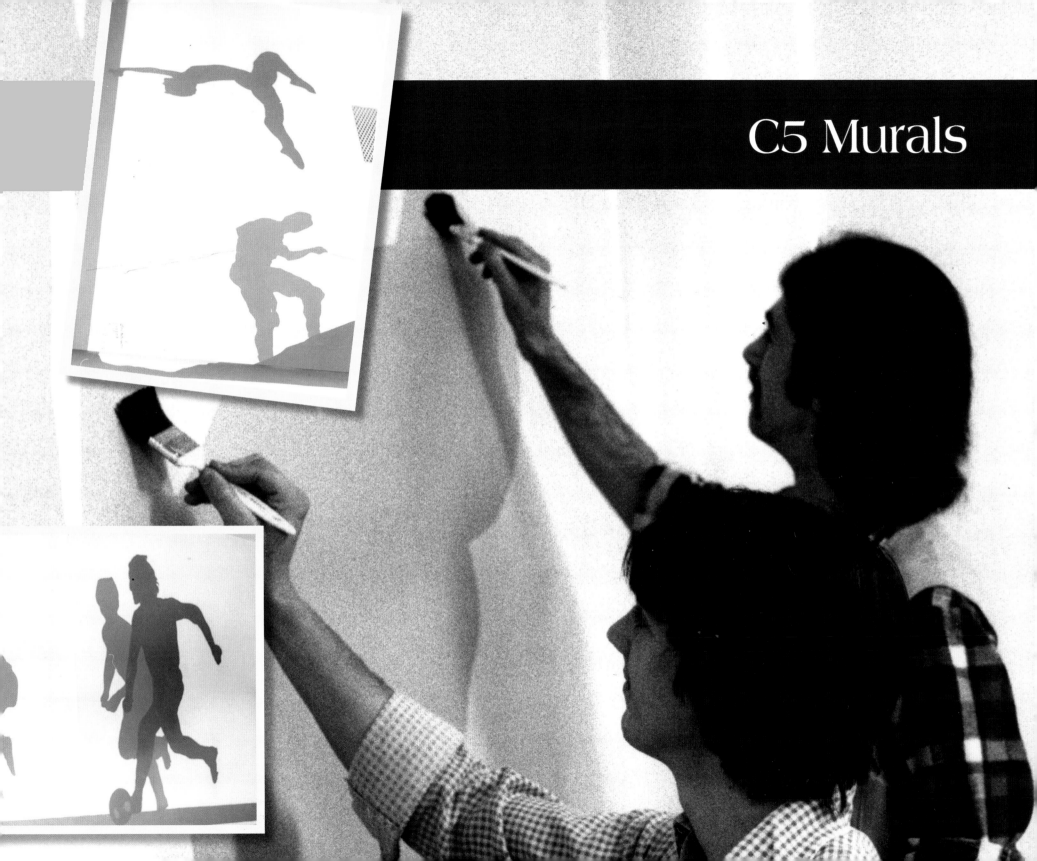

C5 Murals

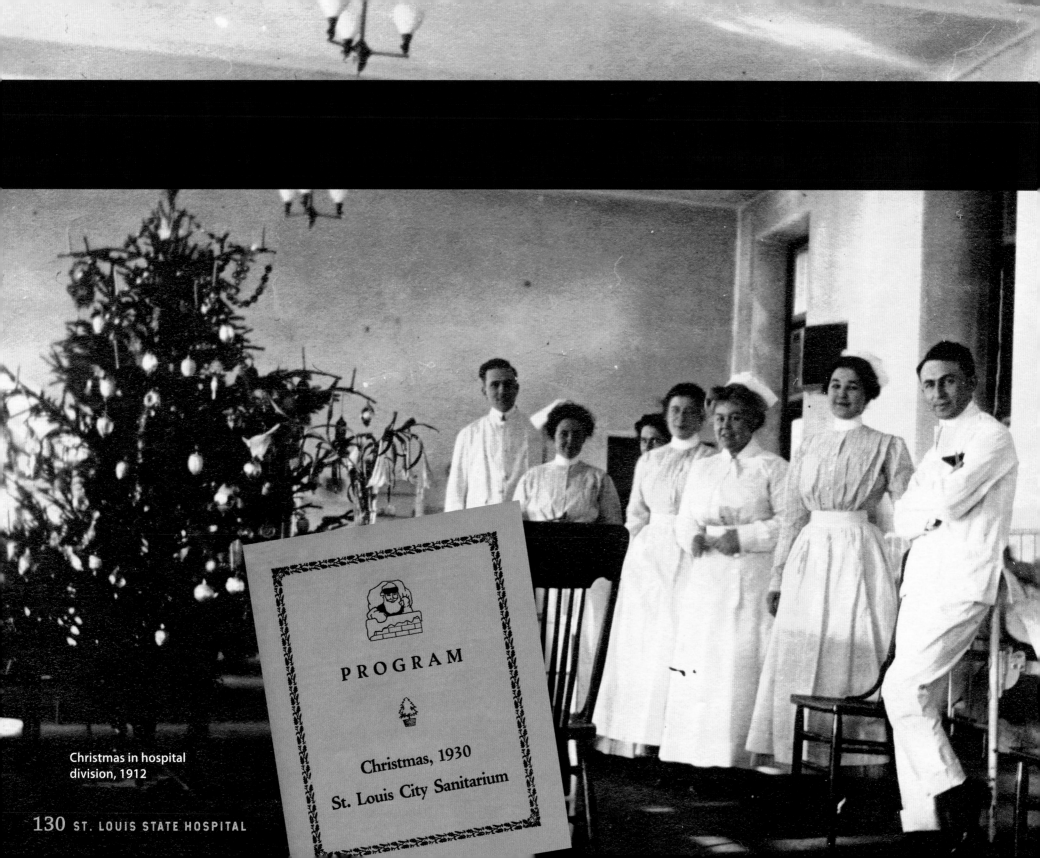

Christmas in hospital
division, 1912

PROGRAM

Christmas, 1930
St. Louis City Sanitarium

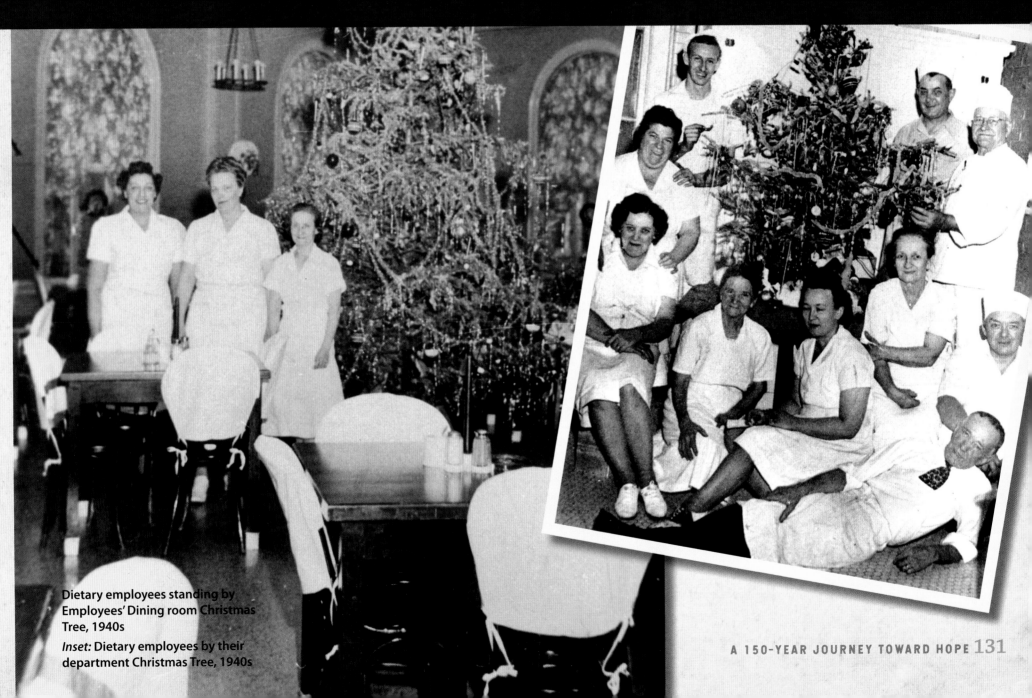

Christmas Through the Years

Dietary employees standing by Employees' Dining room Christmas Tree, 1940s

Inset: Dietary employees by their department Christmas Tree, 1940s

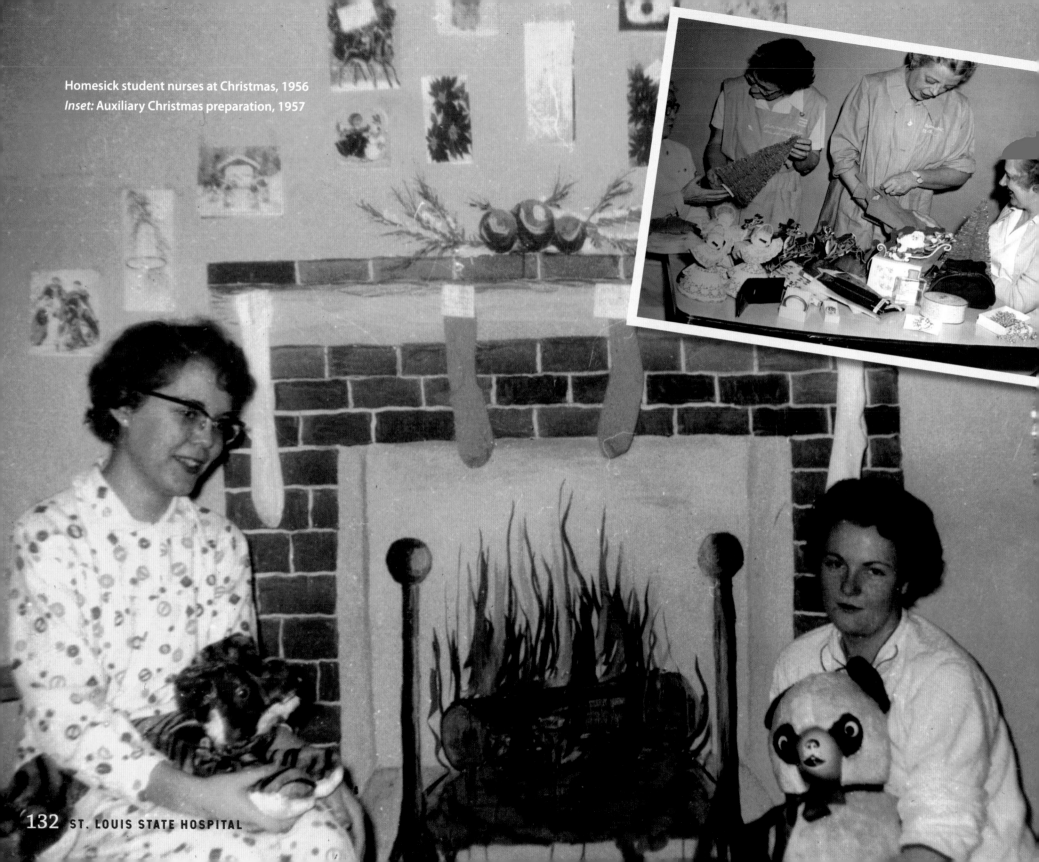

Homesick student nurses at Christmas, 1956
Inset: Auxiliary Christmas preparation, 1957

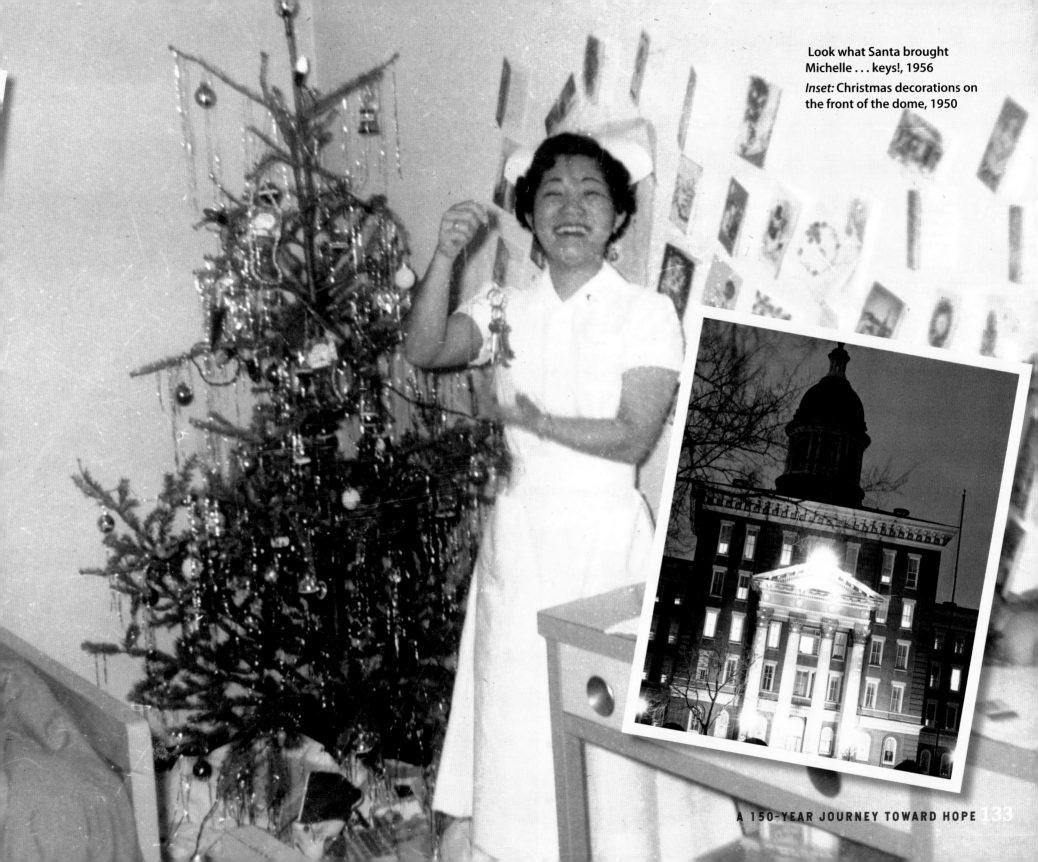

Look what Santa brought Michelle . . . keys!, 1956

Inset: Christmas decorations on the front of the dome, 1950

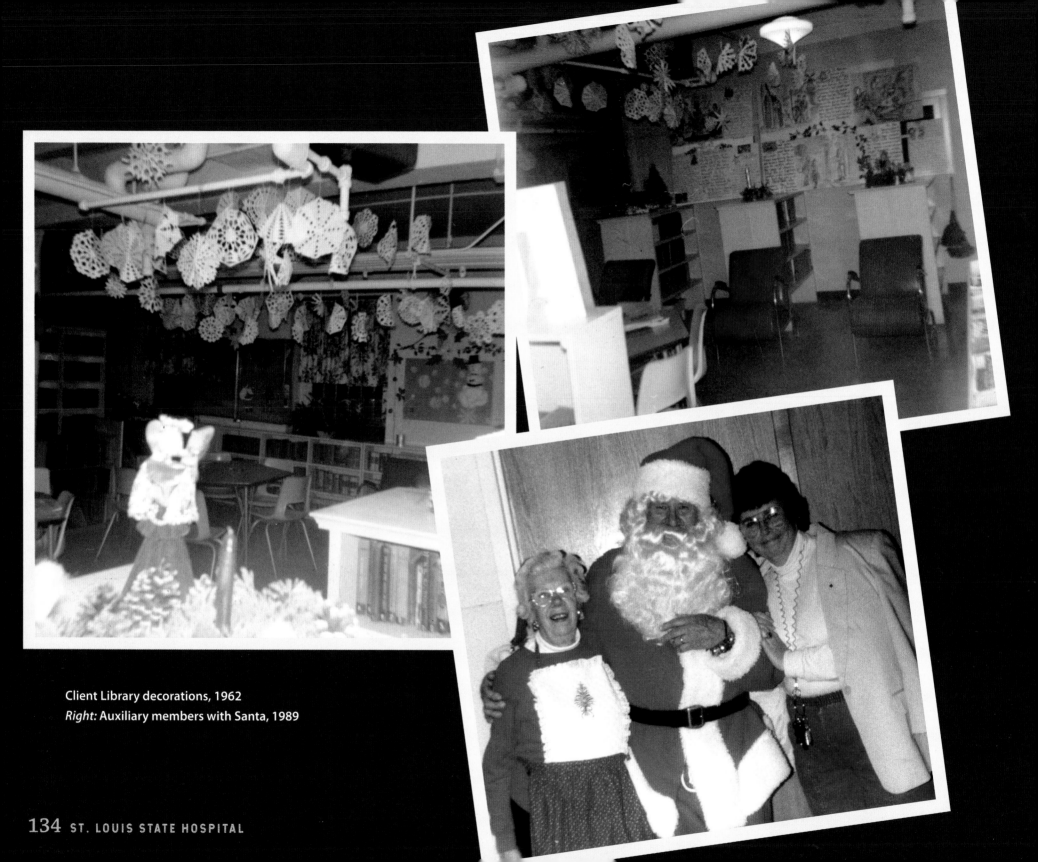

Client Library decorations, 1962
Right: Auxiliary members with Santa, 1989

Psychiatric day care
Christmas trees, 1974

Welcome to C-3
WINTER WONDERLAND
MERRY CHRISMAS and a HAPPY NEW YEAR
FROM THE C-3 FAMILY

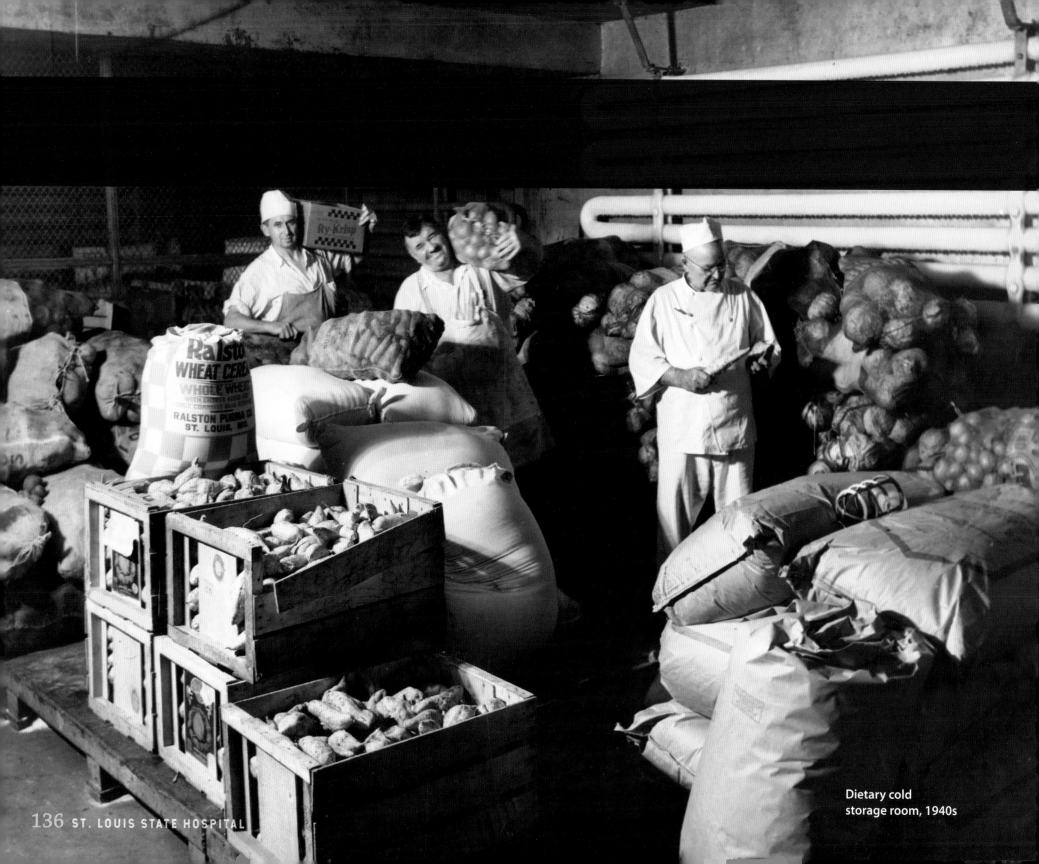

Dietary cold
storage room, 1940s

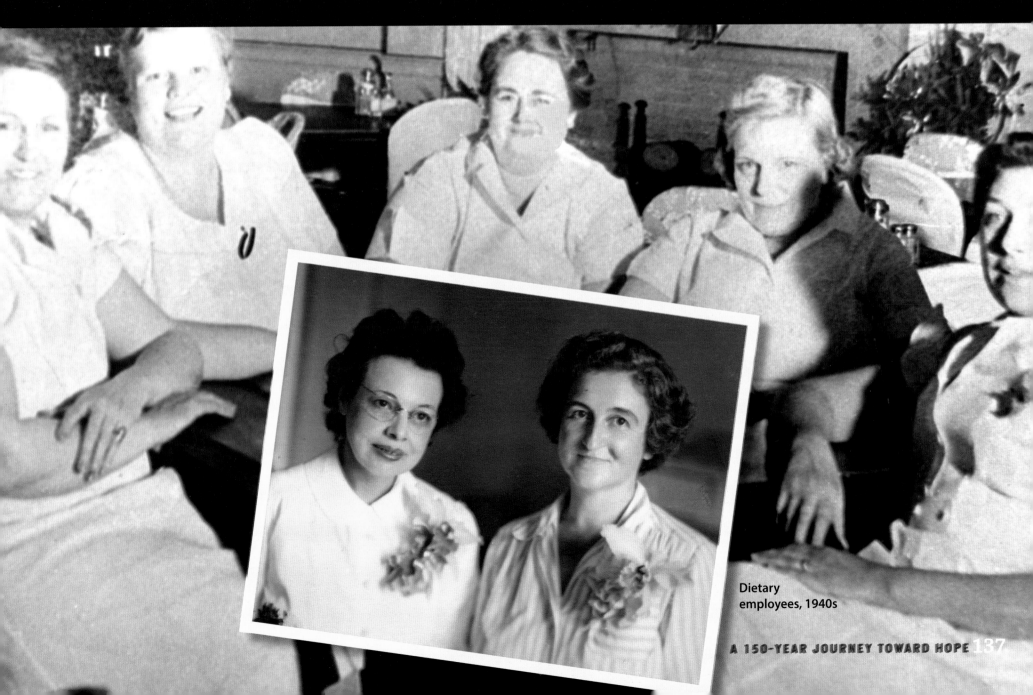

Dietary

Dietary
employees, 1940s

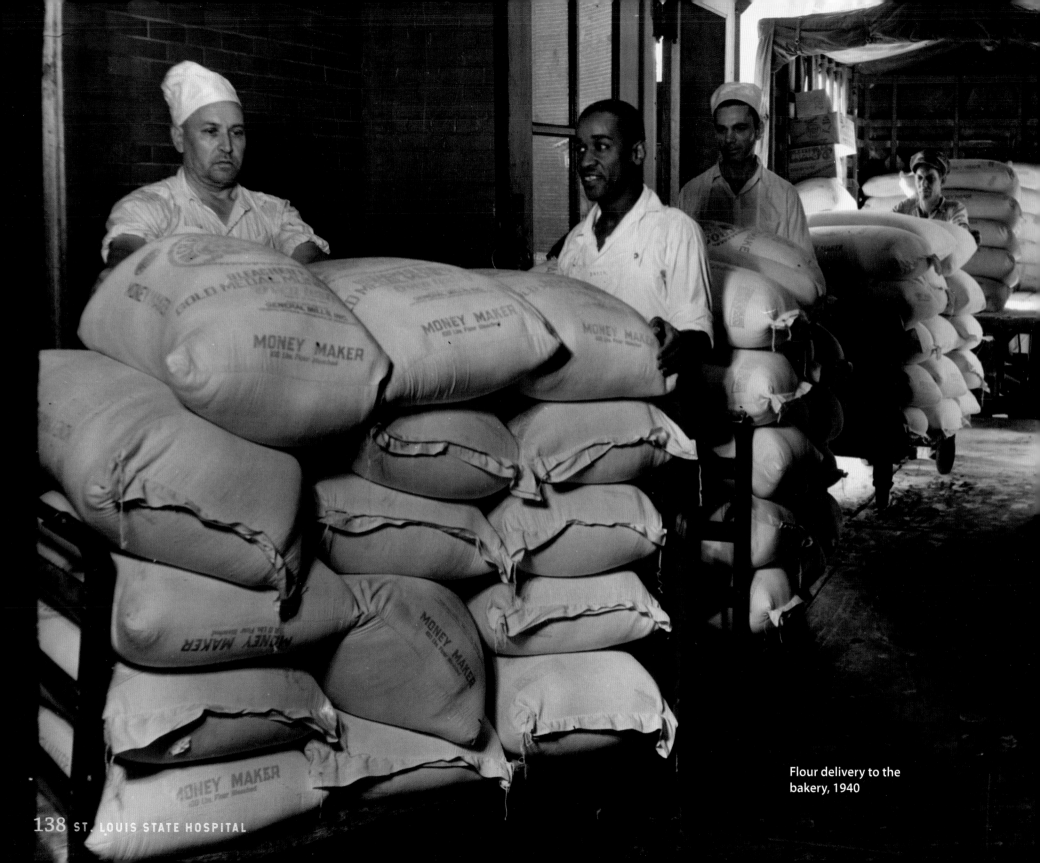

Flour delivery to the bakery, 1940

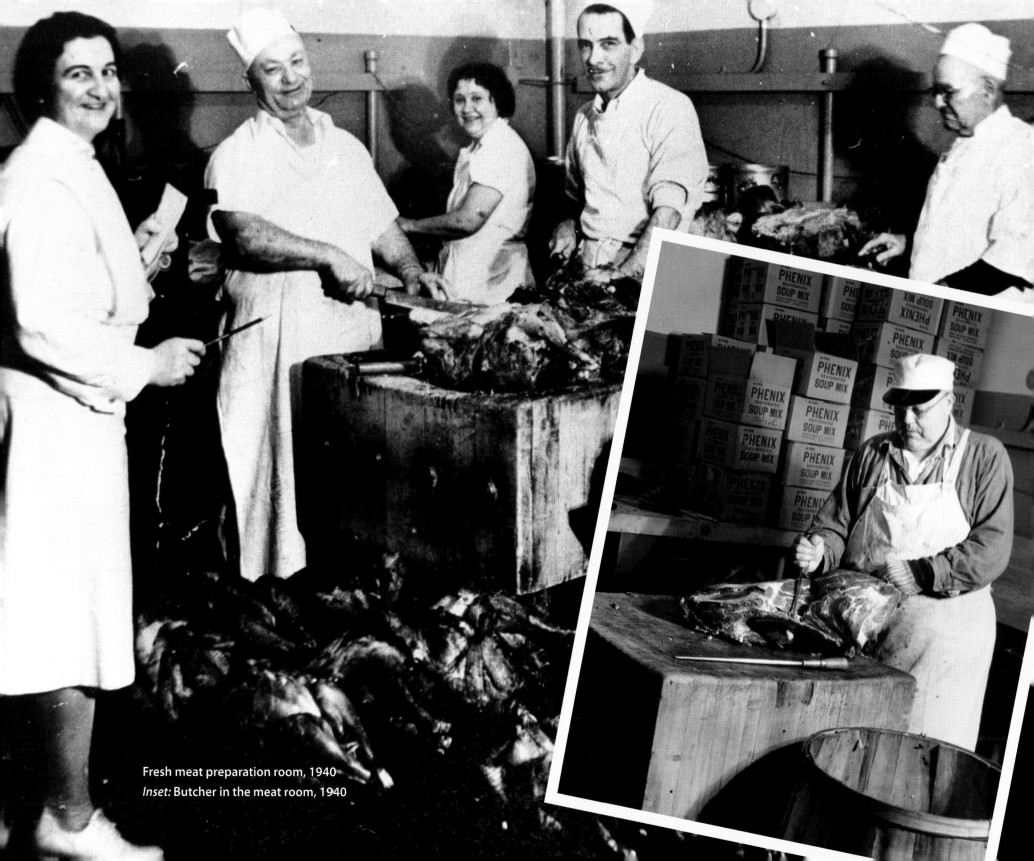

Fresh meat preparation room, 1940
Inset: Butcher in the meat room, 1940

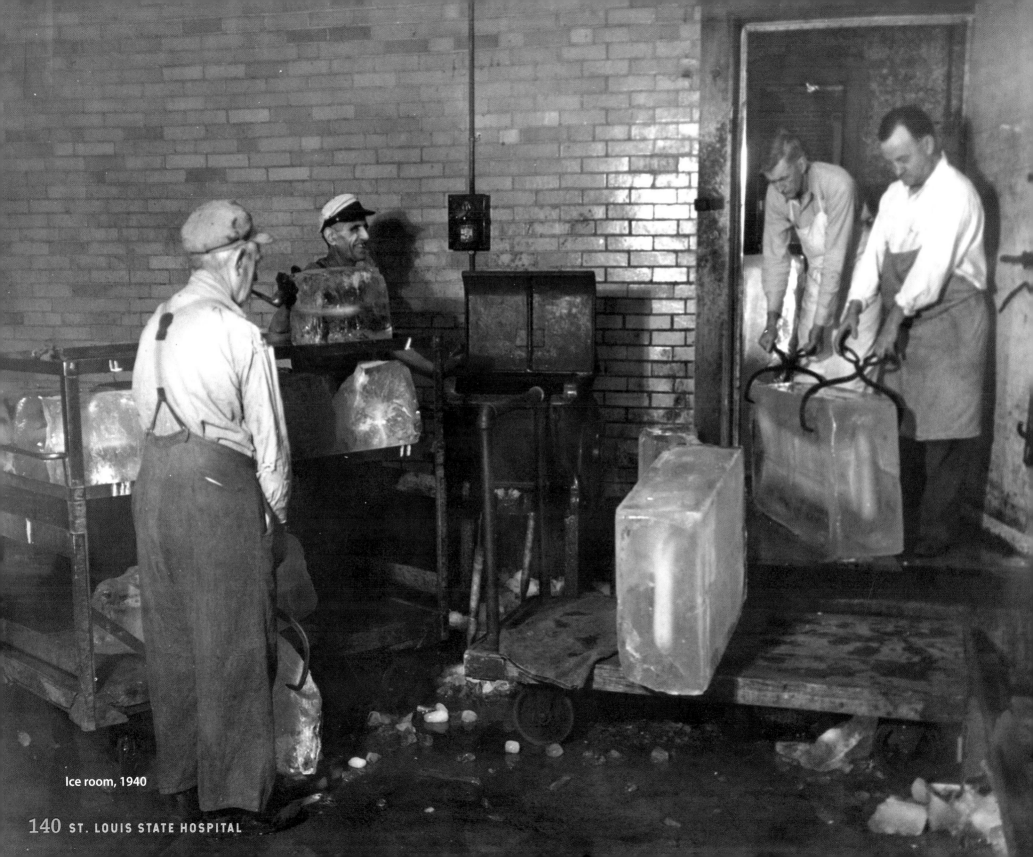

Ice room, 1940

Fresh vegetable preparation room, 1930
Inset: Daily meal preparation, 1940

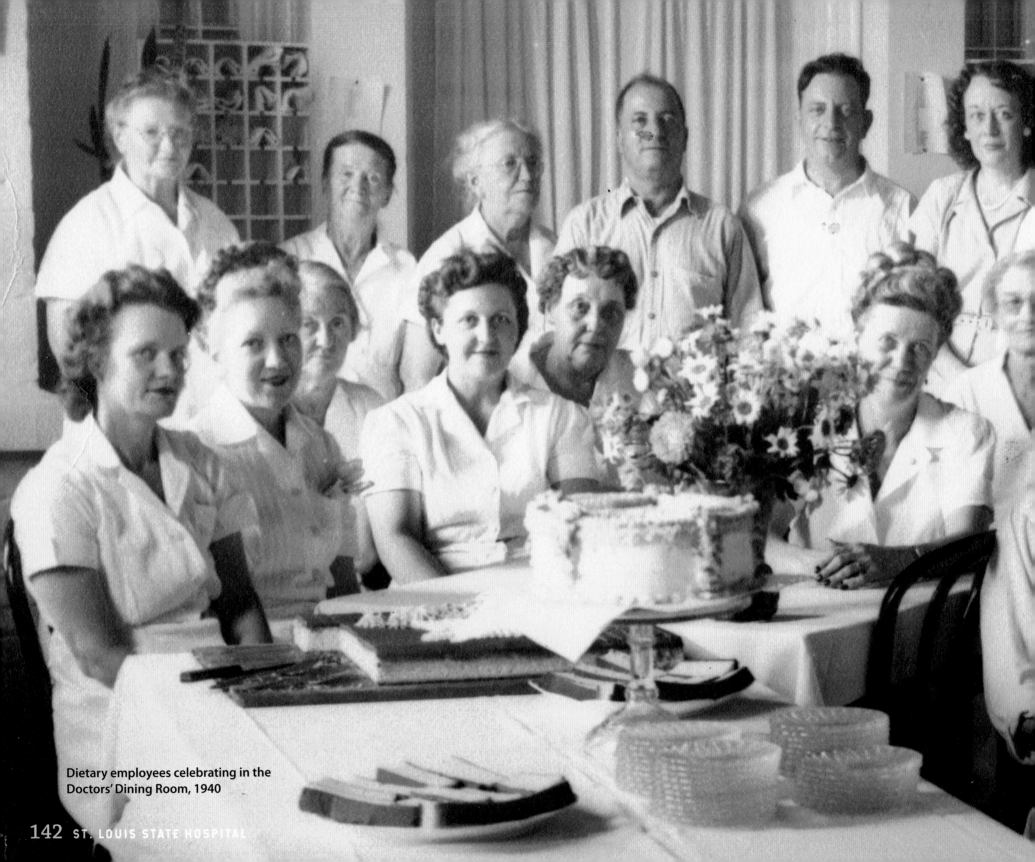

Dietary employees celebrating in the
Doctors' Dining Room, 1940

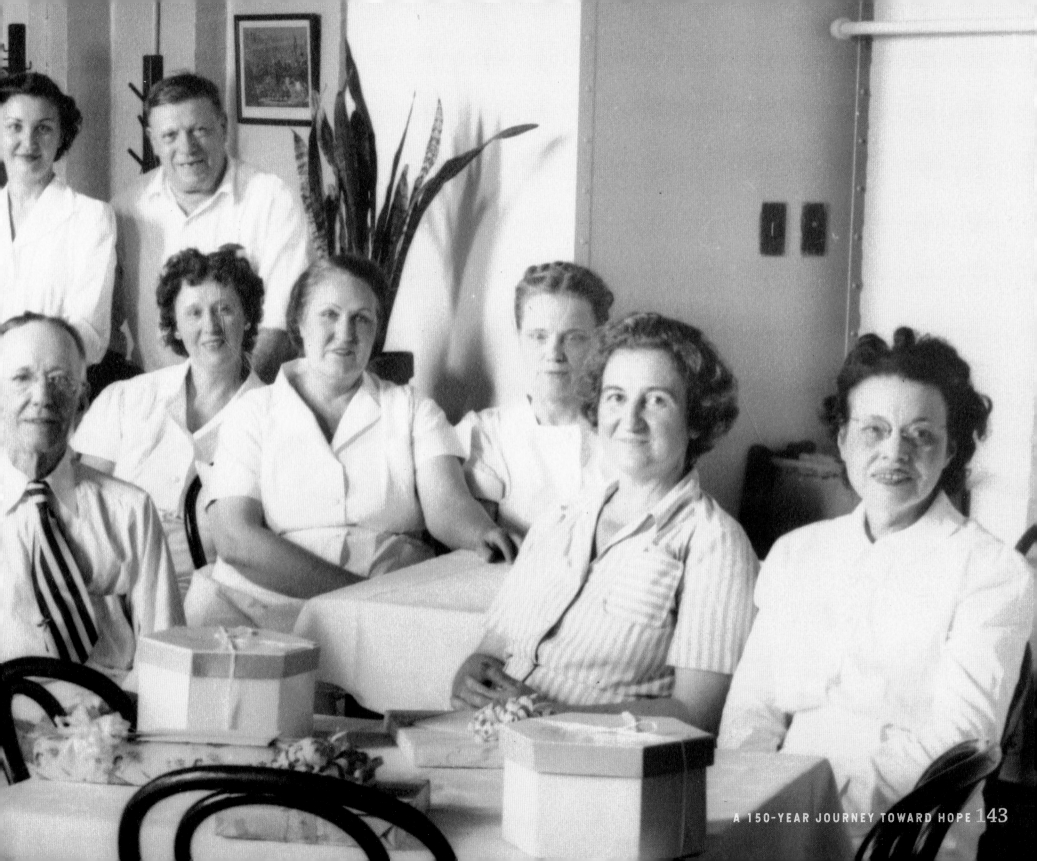

St. Louis County Insane Asylum

Charles Whittlesey Stevens	1869–1872
W.B. Hazard	1872–1873
Jerome K. Bauduy *Dr. Baudy was famous, or infamous depending on the audience, for his progressive views on healthcare for city prostitutes*	1873–1874
E.S. Frazer	1874–1875
Norman DeVere Howard *During the City and County split of 1876, the confusion of which government was in charge of what institution led to an overlap of superintendents.*	1875–1884

St. Louis City Insane Asylum

Charles Whittlesey Stevens *Due to his popularity and kind nature, Dr. Stevens was asked to come back once Dr. Howard finally agreed to leave.*	1876–1877 1884–1886
LeGrand Atwood *Dr. Atwood fought in the Civil War and brought his Confederacy ideology to his time as Superintendent.*	1886–1892

Ernst Mueller	1892–1895
Edward Charles Runge *Dr. Runge spent most of his time bringing civility and deportment back to the "household."*	1895–1904
Henry Skillman Atkins *Dr. Atkins oversaw the expansion of the campus that allowed for a bit of breathing room.*	1904–1910

City Sanitarium

George A. Johns	1911–1923
Charles A. Shumaker	1923–1925
Elbert J. Lee, Jr. *After his downfall from the health department, Dr. Lee enjoyed heckling the Sanitarium through letters to the editor.*	1925–1929
Raymond C. Fagley	1929–1933
George A. Johns	1933–1934
Francis M. Grogan	1934–1941
Louis Hirsch Kohler *By the time he was named superintendent, Dr. Kohler had already been at the San for almost twenty years.*	1941–1943
Walter Moore	1943–1946

Superintendents

St. Louis State Hospital

Louis Hirsch Kohler
Dr. Kohler returned from World War II a Lt. Colonel and picked up where he left off.　　**1946–1964**

Raymond Knowles　　**1965–1969**

J.M. Holden
Dr. Holden, originally from England, was called back home due to a family emergency. So abrupt was his departure that his goodbyes had to be sent via the Employee Bulletin.　　**1969–1970**

Leopold Hofstatter　　**1970–1972**

Patrick Gannon
Dr. Gannon quit in a huff due to his disagreements with state politicians.　　**1972–1976**

Sadashiv Parwatikar
Though of advanced years, Dr. Sam continues to work for the hospital. He credits his health to meditation and a good diet.　　**1976–1978**

John Twiehaus
The first non-medical doctor to take the office.　　**1978–1979**

Milton Fujita
Dr. Fujita was the last medical doctor to serve as superintendent.　　**1979–1988**

Robert O. Muether　　**1988–1989**

Curtis Trager (acting)
Trager "acted" the part for several years until the return of John Twiehaus could happen.　　**1989–1994**

John Twiehaus
Moving to the new, smaller facility brought along a name change and a restructuring of administration leading to the end of superintendents.　　**1994–1997**

"Whilst in a pecuniary point of view I have not found it a 'Bonanza,' but it is an honor to which any man who loves his profession might, with laudable ambition, aspire." —*Dr. E. S. Frazer, 1875*

Index